Evidence-based Dentistry

Guest Editor

MARK V. THOMAS, DMD

DENTAL CLINICS OF NORTH AMERICA

www.dental.theclinics.com

January 2009 • Volume 53 • Number 1

SAUNDERS an imprint of ELSEVIER, Inc.

W.B. SAUNDERS COMPANY
A Division of Elsevier Inc.

1600 John F. Kennedy Boulevard • Suite 1800 • Philadelphia, Pennsylvania 19103-2899

http://www.dental.theclinics.com

DENTAL CLINICS OF NORTH AMERICA Volume 53, Number 1
January 2009 ISSN 0011-8532, ISBN-13: 978-1-4377-0466-2, ISBN-10: 1-4377-0466-2

Editor: John Vassallo; j.vassallo@elsevier.com
Developmental Editor: Donald Mumford

Dental Clinics of North America (ISSN 0011-8532) is published quarterly by Elsevier Inc., 360 Park Avenue South, New York, NY 10010-1710. Months of issue are January, April, July, and October. Business and Editorial Offices: 1600 John F. Kennedy Boulevard, Suite 1800, Philadelphia, PA 19103-2899. Customer Service Office: 11830 Westline Industrial Drive, St. Louis, MO 63146. Periodicals postage paid at New York, NY and additional mailing offices. Subscription prices are $207.00 per year (domestic individuals), $347.00 per year (domestic institutions), $100.00 per year (domestic students/residents), $246.00 per year (Canadian individuals), $437.00 per year (Canadian institutions), $297.00 per year (international individuals), $437.00 per year (international institutions), and $150.00 per year (international and Canadian students/residents). International air speed delivery is included in all *Clinics* subscription prices. All prices are subject to change without notice. **POSTMASTER:** Send address changes to *Dental Clinics of North America*, 11830 Westline Industrial Drive, St. Louis, MO 63146. **Customer Service (orders, claims, online, change of address): Elsevier Periodicals Customer Service, 11830 Westline Industrial Drive, St. Louis, MO 63146. Tel: 1-800-654-2452 (U.S. and Canada). Fax: 314-523-5170. E-mail: journalscustomerservice-usa@elsevier.com (for print support); journalsonlinesupport-usa@elsevier.com (for online support).**

Reprints. For copies of 100 or more, of articles in this publication, please contact the Commercial Reprints Department, Elsevier Inc., 360 Park Avenue South, New York, NY 10010-1710. Tel.: 212-633-3812; Fax: 212-462-1935; E-mail: reprints@elsevier.com.

The *Dental Clinics of North America* is covered in *MEDLINE/PubMed (Index Medicus)*, *Current Contents/Clinical Medicine*, *ISI/BIOMED* and *Clinahl*.

Printed in the United States of America.

Contributors

GUEST EDITOR

MARK V. THOMAS, DMD
Chair, Department of Oral Health Practice; and Chief, Division of Periodontology, University of Kentucky College of Dentistry, Lexington, Kentucky

AUTHORS

JIHAAD ABDUL-MAJID, BS
Dental Student, University of Kentucky College of Dentistry, Lexington, Kentucky

MOHANAD AL-SABBAGH, DDS, MS
Program Director of Graduate Periodontology, Division of Periodontology, University of Kentucky College of Dentistry, Lexington, Kentucky

JAMES D. BADER, DDS, MPH
Research Professor, Operative Dentistry, School of Dentistry, University of North Carolina, Chapel Hill, North Carolina

JEAN BEAUCHAMP, DDS
Private Practice, Clarksville, Tennessee

GEORGE H. BLAKEY, DDS
Clinical Assistant Professor and Residency Program Director, Department of Oral and Maxillofacial Surgery, School of Dentistry, University of North Carolina at Chapel Hill, Chapel Hill, North Carolina

AMANDA BROWN
Division of Periodontology, University of Kentucky College of Dentistry, Lexington, Kentucky

PAGE W. CAUFIELD, DDS, PhD
Professor, Department of Cariology and Comprehensive Care, New York University, College of Dentistry, New York, New York

JAMES J. CRALL, DDS, ScD
Professor and Chair of Pediatric Dentistry, School of Dentistry, University of California Los Angeles, Los Angeles, California

KEVIN J. DONLY, DDS, MS
Professor and Chair, Department of Pediatric Dentistry, Dental School, University of Texas Health Science Center at San Antonio, San Antonio, Texas

ROBERT FEIGAL, DDS, PhD
Professor of Pediatric Dentistry, Department of Preventive Sciences, University of Minnesota, Minneapolis, Minnesota

MARGHERITA FONTANA, DDS, PhD
Associate Professor and Director, Microbial Caries Facility, Oral Health Research Institute; and Director of Predoctoral Education, Department of Preventive and Community Dentistry, Indiana University School of Dentistry, Indianapolis, Indiana

JULIE FRANTSVE-HAWLEY, PhD
Director, Research Institute and Center for Evidence-based Dentistry, American Dental Association, Chicago, Illinois

PAUL A. FUGAZZOTTO, DDS
Private Practice, Milton, Massachusetts

JANE GILLETTE, DDS
Northwest Practice-based REsearch Collaborative in Evidence-based DENTistry, Bozeman, Montana

BARBARA GOOCH, DMD, MPH
Dental Officer, Division of Oral Health, National Center for Health Promotion and Disease Prevention, Centers for Disease Control and Prevention, Atlanta, Georgia

ERSHAL HARRISON, DMD
Assistant Professor, Division of Comprehensive Care, University of Kentucky College of Dentistry, Lexington, Kentucky

RICHARD H. HAUG, DDS
The Provost's Distinguished Service Professor and Executive Associate Dean, University of Kentucky College of Dentistry, Lexington, Kentucky

AMID ISMAIL, BDS, MPH, MBA, DrPH
Professor, University of Michigan, School of Dentistry, Ann Arbor, Michigan

WILLIAM KOHN, DDS
Associate Director of Science, Division of Oral Health, National Center for Health Promotion and Disease Prevention, Centers for Disease Control and Prevention, Atlanta, Georgia

ROBERT E. KOVARIK, DMD, MS
Associate Professor, Department of Oral Health Science, University of Kentucky College of Dentistry, Lexington, Kentucky

JOSEPH D. MATTHEWS, DDS, MSc
Adjunct Faculty Member, University of New Mexico, School of Medicine; AEG Residency, Los Alamos, New Mexico

PATRICIA NIHILL, DMD
Division of Comprehensive Care, University of Kentucky College of Dentistry, Lexington, Kentucky

FONDA G. ROBINSON, DMD
Division of Restorative Dentistry, University of Kentucky College of Dentistry, Lexington, Kentucky

MARK SIEGAL, DDS, MPH
Chief, Ohio Department of Health, Bureau of Oral Health Services, Columbus, Ohio

RICHARD SIMONSEN, DDS, MS
Professor and Dean, Midwestern University, College of Dental Medicine, Glendale, Arizona

SHARON E. STRAUS, MD
Faculty of Medicine, University of Toronto, Toronto, Ontario, Canada

MARK V. THOMAS, DMD
Chair, Department of Oral Health Practice; and Chief, Division of Periodontology, University of Kentucky College of Dentistry, Lexington, Kentucky

ROBERT J. WEYANT, DMD, DrPH
Professor and Chair, Department of Dental Public Health and Information Management, School of Dental Medicine, University of Pittsburgh, Pittsburgh, Pennsylvania

RAYMOND P. WHITE, DDS
Dalton L. McMichael Professor and Residency Program Director, Department of Oral and Maxillofacial Surgery, School of Dentistry, University of North Carolina at Chapel Hill, Chapel Hill, North Carolina

MARK S. WOLFF, DDS, PhD
Professor and Chair, Department of Cariology and Comprehensive Care, New York University College of Dentistry, New York, New York

DOUGLAS A. YOUNG, DDS, MS, MBA
Associate Professor, Department of Dental Practice, University of the Pacific, San Francisco, San Francisco, California

Contents

> Evidence-based health care seeks to base clinical practice and decision-making on best evidence, while allowing for modifications because of patient preferences and individual clinical situations. Dentistry has been slow to embrace this discipline, but this is changing. In the Graduate Periodontology Program (GPP) of the University of Kentucky, an evidence-based clinical curriculum was implemented in 2004. The tools of evidence-based health care (EBHC) were used to create evidence-based protocols to guide clinical decision-making by faculty and residents. The program was largely successful, although certain challenges were encountered. As a result of the positive experience with the GPP, the college is implementing a wider program in which evidence-based protocols will form the basis for all patient care and clinical education in the predoctoral clinics. A primary component of this is a computerized risk assessment tool that will aid in clinical decision-making. Surveys of alumni of the periodontal graduate program show that the EBHC program has been effective in changing practice patterns, and similar follow-up studies are planned to assess the effectiveness of the predoctoral EBHC program.

> This article presents personal observations on how the concept of evidence-based dentistry is faring in the profession. It considers how the dental profession's concept of evidence has matured, how evidence-based dentistry was originally envisioned, how it is currently embodied, and what its prospects might be for the immediate future. Evidence-based dentistry began in the profession approximately 2 decades ago, initiated by the appearance of the first systematic reviews on dental topics in the late 1980s. The emergence of the concept of evidence-based dentistry—and its fundamental construct, the systematic review—marks what can be considered a fundamental shift in how the dental knowledge base has grown and developed over time.

> Evidence-based medicine requires the integration of best research evidence with the clinician's expertise and the patient's unique values and circumstances. One of the most important issues in deciding what course of treatment to select is balancing the potential risks and benefits of treatment. A framework for evidence-based decision-making includes

formulating the clinical question and then retrieving, appraising, and considering the applicability of the evidence to the patient. It is the duty of all health care providers to reduce patient risk by selecting appropriate therapies and informing patients of unavoidable risks.

Dentistry over the last 100 years has been characterized by improved approaches to education and practice. Parallel to trends in the field of medicine as a whole, dentistry is moving toward evidence-based practices. The goal of evidence-based dentistry is the assurance, through reference to high-quality evidence, that care provided is optimal for the patient and that treatment options are presented in a manner that allows for fully informed consent. As we transition toward broad-based use of evidence-based dentistry approaches in clinical practice, many dental offices will benefit from a better understanding of how evidence-based dentistry can improve patient outcomes. This article lists the likely benefits evidence-based dentistry can provide to patients, staff, and dentists when routinely adopted in daily practice.

Dentinal hypersensitivity is a common dental complaint, especially in periodontal patients. It is believed to be mediated by a hydrodynamic mechanism in which various stimuli result in increased fluid flow in dentinal tubules, thereby generating action potentials in associated nerve fibers. Although it is often perceived as mild discomfort by the patient, it can be severe. A variety of interventions has been used, although few have been subjected to rigorous study. This article surveys those in-office treatments that are available, and suggests directions for research so that clinicians may treat patients based on best evidence. Until such evidence is available, it seems prudent to employ therapies that are least likely to cause harm and are reversible.

This article reviews the evidence regarding the effectiveness of various patient-applied interventions for dentinal hypersensitivity. Self-applied treatments are popular because they are both economical and easy to use. The disadvantages include compliance, difficulty to deliver to specific sites, slow onset of action, and the requirement for continuous use. Conflicting research findings make it difficult for the practitioner to determine which self-applied product to advise patients to use. There are a number of issues that have plagued research in this area, including the lack of standardization of stimulus testing and inadequate sample size. The evidence is insufficient to permit the development of evidence-based guidelines for the treatment of dentinal hypersensitivity.

This article reviews the current use of amalgam versus resin composite in posterior restorations and the evidence-base for choosing between these two treatment options. While much research has been published on the issue of the clinical use of amalgam versus resin composite, there are several issues that limit the true evidence-base on the subject. Furthermore, while the majority of published studies on posterior composites would seem to indicate equivalent clinical performance of resin composite to amalgam restorations, the studies that should be weighted much more heavily (randomized controlled trials) do not support the slant of the rest of the literature. As part of an evidence-based approach to private practice, clinicians need to be aware of the levels of evidence in the literature and need to properly inform patients of the true clinical outcomes that are associated with the use of amalgam versus resin composite for posterior restorations, so that patients are themselves making informed decisions about their dental care.

The American Association of Oral and Maxillofacial Surgeons (AAOMS) has been at the forefront of formal evidence-based dentistry with such projects as the *Parameters of Care: Clinical Practice Guidelines for Oral and Maxillofacial Surgeons*, the AAOMS Outcomes Assessment Program, the AAOMS Third Molar Clinical Trial, and the AAOMS "White Paper on Third Molar Data." This article reviews these evidence-based resources to provide a consensus of opinion for the management of the third molar.

Single-tooth replacement may be effected through various methods, including the use of a resin-bonded fixed partial denture, a conventional fixed partial denture, and a single implant-supported crown. Although the introduction of newer therapeutic modalities, surgical and restorative techniques, and restorative materials has significantly expanded available treatment options, a greater demand is now placed on the diagnostic and treatment planning acumen of the clinician. The questions confronting each clinician are when to apply each treatment modality and how to use these therapeutic approaches to their maximum benefit for the patient. This article focuses on the factors that should be considered when making such clinical decisions and offers a framework within which to formulate appropriate treatment algorithms.

This article presents evidence-based clinical recommendations for use of pit-and-fissure sealants developed by an expert panel convened by the American Dental Association (ADA) Council on Scientific Affairs. The panel addressed the following clinical questions. Under what circumstances should sealants be placed to prevent caries? Does placing sealants over early (noncavitated) lesions prevent progression of the lesion? Are there conditions that favor the placement of resin-based versus glass ionomer cement sealants in terms of retention or caries prevention? Are there any techniques that could improve sealants' retention and effectiveness in caries prevention? Staff of the ADA Division of Science conducted a MEDLINE search to identify systematic reviews and clinical studies published after the identified systematic reviews.

Dental caries is a dietary and host-modified biofilm disease process, transmissible early in life that, if left untreated, will cause destruction of dental hard tissues. If allowed to progress, the disease will result in the development of caries lesions on tooth surfaces, which initially are noncavitated (eg, white spots), and eventually can progress to cavitation. The "medical model," where the etiologic disease-driving agents are balanced against protective factors, in combination with risk assessment, offers the possibility of patient-centered disease prevention and management before there is irreversible damage done to the teeth. This article discusses how to use evidence supporting risk assessment and management strategies for the caries process.

RELATED INTEREST

Oral and Maxillofacial Surgery Clinics of North America November 2008 (Vol. 20, No. 4)
Head and Neck Manifestations of Systemic Disorders
Sidney L. Bourgeois, Jr., DDS, *Guest Editor*

THE CLINICS ARE NOW AVAILABLE ONLINE!

Access your subscription at:
www.theclinics.com

Preface

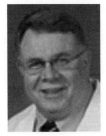

Mark V. Thomas, DMD
Guest Editor

Many years ago, while a graduate student in periodontology, I attended a presentation by the prominent Swedish academician Dr. Jan Lindhe. I had attended many presentations on periodontology, but Lindhe's presentation was different. Rather than speaking of his personal clinical experiences and philosophy, he simply asked a series of questions (eg, "How much attached gingiva is required for gingival health?") and attempted to use literature to answer them. It was such a simple and obvious strategy: the use of evidence to guide our clinical decisions! But it seemed radical and transformative, simply because it was done so rarely at the time.

Every period in history is informed by a *Zeitgeist* or "spirit of the age." The current period is no different. In 21st century health care, the unifying concept may be evidence. Evidence-based health care (EBHC) appears to be a simple idea: doing what works as determined by the evidence. Although the term "evidence-based health care" was not in use at the time I heard Dr. Lindhe's presentation, he was modeling the techniques of EBHC.

EBHC has the potential to transform health care. It can reduce medical errors, improve patient outcomes, and control health care costs. Porter and Teisberg,[1] in their influential text "Redefining Health Care," argue that health care providers and organizations should compete on creating value for the patient. This value is achieved by assessing and improving patient-centered outcomes (which is made possible by basing clinical decisions upon the best evidence) and making these outcomes (another form of evidence) available to consumers (patients).

Of course, there are many gaps in our evidence, as pointed out by detractors of the EBHC movement. They have many concerns, the most compelling of which are related to the validity or integrity of the evidence. Obviously, recommendations can be no better than the evidence upon which they are based. And the evidence is always imperfect. Even more problematic is that evidence often is lacking or insufficient to permit the creation of evidence-based guidelines. But this is changing. Databases, such as the Cochrane Library (http://www.cochrane.org/), now have a considerable number of high-quality dental reviews, and the number is increasing dramatically.

Dent Clin N Am 53 (2009) xiii–xv
doi:10.1016/j.cden.2008.11.005
0011-8532/08/$ – see front matter © 2009 Elsevier Inc. All rights reserved.

dental.theclinics.com

More must be done, however. If EBHC is to realize its promise, it will require effort on the part of three constituencies: the creators of evidence, the compilers of evidence, and the users of evidence. The creators must conduct well-designed clinical trials of sufficient power to permit valid inferences to be drawn from their results. The compilers must act as "honest brokers" in synthesizing this evidence in the form of high-quality systematic reviews that are easily accessed by end-users. Lastly, the users must appraise the evidence and apply it in the service of individual patients. Obviously, many clinicians belong to all three groups.

The contributors to this issue all share a commitment to the principles and practice of evidence-based health care. They approach this subject from a variety of viewpoints. There are reports on educational initiatives, in which the principles of EBHC are used to enhance dental curricula, examples of best practices based on high-level evidence, and several examples of how to proceed when high-quality evidence is lacking. Readers will find a diverse selection of EBHC topics within this issue. It is hoped that this disparate collection of articles will provide the stimulus for further reading in the field.

Readers desiring further information will find a number of attractive resources available to them. *Evidence-Based Medicine: How to Practice and Teach EBM* by Straus and colleagues is foremost.[2] This small, easily read volume is in its third edition and is an overview of the tools of EBM. A more comprehensive text is the *Users' Guides to the Medical Literature* by Guyatt and colleagues.[3] This book provides a more thorough discussion of many EBHC topics and is recommended to the reader seeking in-depth knowledge. I also recommend *Evidence-based Dentistry: Managing Information for Better Practice* by Richards and colleagues.[4] I had the pleasure of reviewing this work recently and found it to be a succinct survey of EBHC as applied to dentistry. Lastly, I would recommend Elwood's *Critical Appraisal of Epidemiological Studies and Clinical Trials* for a comprehensive examination of the techniques used to appraise evidence.[5] Much of the peer-reviewed literature now contains systematic reviews and meta-analyses, and these can be found (to varying degrees) in most scholarly journals. *The Journal of Evidence-Based Dental Practice* is of particular interest. The September 2008 issue of that journal, entitled "Evidence-Based Champion Conference" was jointly sponsored by the American Dental Association and the *Journal of Evidence-Based Dental Practice*.[6] This issue is highly recommended as an overview on the state of the art and suggests the importance of EBHC from the perspective of organized dentistry.

The pieces are now in place to allow the transformation of health care. We have better evidence and the electronic means to search for and access it, and we are developing a cadre of young clinicians who are being taught that their clinical decisions should be based on the best evidence. Evidence-based medicine, with its foundational sciences of clinical epidemiology and biostatistics, will transform health care in the 21st century as thoroughly as molecular biology transformed health care in the 20th century. It will be an exciting time.

Mark V. Thomas, DMD
Department of Oral Health Practice
Division of Periodontology
University of Kentucky College of Dentistry
800 Rose Street, Room M-122
Lexington, KY 40536-0297, USA

E-mail address:
mvthom0@email.uky.edu (M.V. Thomas)

REFERENCES

1. Porter ME, Teisberg EO. Redefining health care: creating value-based competition on results. Boston (MA): Harvard Business School Press; 2006.
2. Straus SE, Richardon WS, Glasziou P, et al. Evidence-based medicine: how to practice and teach EBM. 3rd edition. Edinburgh: Elsevier Churchill Livingstone; 2005.
3. Guyatt G, Rennie D. Users' guides to the medical literature. Chicago: AMA Press; 2002.
4. Richards D, Clarkson J, Matthews D, et al. Evidence-based dentistry: managing information for better practice. London: Quintessence; 2008.
5. Elwood M. Critical appraisal of epidemiological studies and clinical trials. New York: Oxford; 1998.
6. Journal of Evidence-Based Dental Practice 2008;8(3):113–208.

Evidence-Based Curriculum Reform: The Kentucky Experience

Mark V. Thomas, DMD[a],*, Fonda G. Robinson, DMD[b], Patricia Nihill, DMD[c]

KEYWORDS

• Evidence-based • Dentistry • Teaching • Curriculum

Evidence-based medicine (EBM) has been described as "the conscientious, explicit, and judicious use of current best evidence in making decision about the care of individual patients."[1] One of the defining characteristics of EBM is that formal processes are used for assessing the reliability of the clinical evidence used to inform clinical decisions.[2] The drivers of the EBM movement have been the need for reliable information by busy clinicians, the shortcomings of traditional sources of information (eg, textbooks), the availability of online databases that serve as repositories of this information, the limited time available to physicians to access information, and the electronic technology that has made searching the databases a simple matter. Another enabling factor is the maturation of clinical epidemiology as a discipline and its application to decision-making in health care.[3] Currently pressure has increased to improve patient outcomes, reduce medical errors, make health care more accessible, and reduce medical expenses.[4] Ample evidence shows that medical decision-making is often inconsistent and not based on best evidence or practices.[5,6] EBM may help alleviate these problems and contribute to improving the quality and consistency of health care.

After a slow start, EBM is beginning to exert a profound effect on health care. Dentistry has been slower than medicine to adopt evidence-based strategies, but this is changing. Recently, the American Dental Association (ADA) held two evidence-based dentistry (EBD) conferences to promote this concept.[7–10] The ADA hopes to create a cadre of "EBD Champions" who will, it is hoped, return to their communities or institutions and promote EBD and its many benefits. Because the conceptual foundation and tools of EBM and EBD are the same, this article uses the more inclusive term *evidence-based health care* (EBHC) to refer to these concepts.

[a] Department of Oral Health Practice, Division of Periodontology, University of Kentucky College of Dentistry, 800 Rose Street, Room M-122, Lexington, KY 40536-0297, USA
[b] Division of Restorative Dentistry, University of Kentucky College of Dentistry, 800 Rose Street, Lexington, KY 40536-0297, USA
[c] Division of Comprehensive Care, University of Kentucky College of Dentistry, 800 Rose Street, Lexington, KY 40536-0297, USA
* Corresponding author.
E-mail address: mvthom0@uky.edu (M. Thomas).

Dent Clin N Am 53 (2009) 1–13
doi:10.1016/j.cden.2008.10.002
0011-8532/08/$ – see front matter © 2009 Elsevier Inc. All rights reserved.

EBHC consists of five steps, which have been described in greater detail elsewhere:[11]

1. Convert the need for clinical information into an answerable question
2. Find and rank the best evidence with which to answer the question
3. Critically appraise the evidence for validity, impact, and applicability
4. Integrate this evidence with clinical expertise and the patient's unique circumstances and preferences
5. Evaluate effectiveness and efficiency in executing steps 1 through 4

The first step is to convert the clinician's need for information into an answerable question. This question may be more "background," which is concerned with a gap in general knowledge about a condition, diagnostic test, or intervention. A dental example might be "Does oral bisphosphonate therapy have an effect on implant survival?" Questions concerning the specific management of a patient may be termed *foreground questions*. For example, one might ask, "In a 45-year-old female smoker with osteoporosis, what is the risk for implant loss?" The relative need for background or foreground information varies with clinical experience.[11] When dentists have little experience with the condition of interest, more background information is required, which is the situation for third-year medical or dental students (or experienced clinicians who are confronted with an unusual clinical condition). When dentists have more experience, they are more likely to require focused information relating to specific patient management issues (eg, the situation faced by a second-year resident or an experienced clinician).

The second step is finding the best evidence with which to answer this question and then ranking it according to the hierarchy of evidence shown in **Fig. 1**. Individual studies are at the bottom of this pyramid, whereas databases or repositories in which syntheses of evidence may be located (eg, the Cochrane Library) are somewhat higher. Synoptic journals are next, followed by computerized clinical decision support systems, which are capable of assimilating the data for a given patient and suggesting interventions (or further diagnostic tests) based on best evidence.

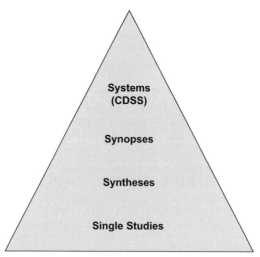

Fig. 1. Hierarchy of evidence. (*Adapted from* Straus SE, Richardon WS, Glasziou P, et al. Evidence-based medicine: how to practice and teach EBM. Edinburgh: Elsevier Churchill Livingstone; 2005; with permission.)

Ideally, there would be a seamless link between the clinical decision support system and the patient's electronic health record, so that suggestions regarding the patient's diagnosis and treatment would be made in real time as data is entered into the chart. This system would be automatically updated with the latest best evidence as it became available. Obviously, these systems are not in general use, but the soundness of this approach has been shown, particularly in the area of prescribing multiple medications for hospitalized or geriatric patients. To date, the applications with the most immediate usefulness have been those that promote guideline adherence and alert providers to drug interactions or treatment omissions.[12] Examples include computer provider order entry systems combined with clinical decision support systems, which have been shown to improve patient safety through reducing the incidence of adverse drug interactions.[13,14]

The third step of the classical EBHC process is critical appraisal of the evidence. Evidence must be screened for validity, impact, and clinical applicability. Of particular interest is the concept of *external validity*. A study is said to possess external validity when it can provide "unbiased inferences regarding a target population (beyond the subjects in the study)."[15] This finding is a function of the study population vis-à-vis the research hypothesis. If a study on melanoma risk factors recruited only Caucasian women, the conclusions generated may not apply to African American men, who experience a much lower incidence of this cancer.[16] Populations differ and these differences may have an important effect on study outcomes.

Another example of this population difference is the prevalence of a genotype associated with severe periodontitis.[17–19] The genotype is present in approximately 30% of individuals of northern European descent, but a study in a Chinese population found a prevalence of only 2.3%.[20] These differences must be considered when extrapolating the results of a study to a more general (or different) population than the study sample.

The impact of the evidence can be measured by the size of the treatment effect for therapeutic interventions. This effect can be reported in a number of ways, depending on the intervention. For example, the relative risk reduction is useful in describing the protective effect of a therapy (eg, fluoride varnish). For other types of interventions, a relative benefit increase may be more appropriate. One particularly useful concept is the number needed to treat, which is the number of patients that must be treated with the therapy in question to prevent one additional bad outcome (however that is defined).

The impact of a diagnostic test can be assessed through examining the sensitivity, specificity, positive predictive value, and negative predictive value. Finally, the intervention must be clinically applicable to each unique patient. This critical appraisal is at the heart of the EBHC concept and is, to a large extent, what Straus and colleagues[11] refer to as "doing" EBHC. The basic process is often referred to as "critical thinking" in academic health care, and it is a critical competency for clinicians, regardless of discipline.

EBHC has begun to appear in the dental curriculum.[21–23] These EBHC experiences often consist of sending students to the library, where they conduct searches of the primary literature on some assigned topic and then critique the papers found. These worthwhile exercises are performed with the laudable goal of fostering "critical thinking." Students are assumed to carry these skills into practice and used to improve patient outcomes.

Unfortunately, busy clinicians have insufficient time to perform lengthy analyses of the primary literature. Lack of time is cited as one of the drivers of the EBHC movement. Sackett and colleagues [24] originally envisioned EBHC as a quick and efficient way to access best evidence and found that making evidence readily available increased the likelihood that this evidence would be used in making clinical decisions.

Obviously, critically analyzing one randomized controlled trial is an intellectually valuable exercise for health care students. As valuable as this exercise is, however, it is incomplete because it does not really give students a good model for incorporating EBHC into clinical practice. What is needed is quick access to robust information, such as that supplied by systematic reviews or meta-analyses like those found in the Cochrane Library or similar sources.[25,26] Only when these reviews are not available should a search of the primary literature be required. Unfortunately, most clinicians will have neither the time nor the inclination to perform their own reviews (and may be hard-pressed to conduct searches for even single articles).

In this regard, a useful distinction might be made between "doers" of EBHC and "users" of EBHC. Straus and colleagues[11] point out that clinicians may shift back and forth between the "using" and "doing" modes. They note that "while some clinicians may want to become proficient in practicing all five steps of EBHC, many others would instead prefer to focus on becoming efficient users (and knowledge managers) of evidence."[11] Although students of all health care disciplines must be competent in both "using" and "doing," it seems that they must at least be able to access and use best evidence, which involves different tools and a different approach than "doing" EBHC. University of Kentucky College of Dentistry (UKCD) requires students to be competent in both modes, but has emphasized the "using" mode in clinical protocols and education, because they believe it to be the mode most likely to be used by most graduates.

A small group at the UKCD became interested in using EBHC principles to enhance curriculum and clinical services. This article presents a brief review of UKCD's initial experiences in implementing this initiative. Although they are in the process of creating a predoctoral clinical curriculum based on the concepts of EBHC, much of their experience has been in the Graduate Periodontology Program. The goal was to fully and seamlessly integrate EBHC into the clinical curriculum. The idea was to make it truly an organic part of the clinical and educational missions of the college, because they believed this was the best way to show the usefulness of EBHC to skeptical students and faculty.

The goal was to use the principles and tools of EBHC to guide clinical decision making through the creation of evidence-based treatment protocols for commonly encountered clinical situations. This information was to be incorporated into didactic coursework and applied in the clinical setting. These clinical protocols were to be easily accessed by students, faculty, and staff. This represents a more holistic and integrated form of EBHC than an individual course devoted to EBHC (although the two approaches are not, of course, mutually exclusive).

Korenstein and colleagues[27] reported a similar program at Mount Sinai School of Medicine, in which EBHC is fully integrated into clinical curricula, including women's health and addiction medicine. The programs have been well received and plans call for expanding this approach into other areas of the curriculum.

TEACHING EVIDENCE-BASED HEALTH CARE

One challenge confronting clinical teachers is how best to incorporate EBHC into the curriculum. Three primary modes of teaching EBHC exist:[11]

1. Role-modeling evidence-based practice
2. Using (and making explicit) the use of evidence in clinical teaching
3. Teaching the skills of EBHC ("doing" EBHC)

The first is the practice of EBHC so that it is seamlessly integrated into the care of patients. The second mode involves learning EBHC principles through integrating research evidence into clinical and didactic teaching so that students can see the evidentiary foundation of their education. The third mode involves teaching the skills of "doing" EBHC, wherein students learn to find and critically appraise the evidence. This step is necessary to develop critical thinking skills and, as importantly, give students the tools needed for lifelong learning.

Efforts have been strongly influenced by those of Sackett, Straus, and their colleagues.[3,11,28] Their experience in implementing EBHC into their clinic is extensive and their insights into what makes for effective (and ineffective) EBHC teaching are invaluable. They have identified several factors associated with success when teaching EBHC:[11]

1. Process is based on clinical decisions
2. Focus is on learners' actual learning needs
3. Passive and active learning are both used in a balanced manner
4. What is already known is connected with "new" knowledge
5. Teacher is explicit about appraisal of evidence
6. EBHC is seamlessly integrated into patient care decisions
7. Provides a foundation and tools for lifelong learning

They suggest that EBHC teaching success occurs when the EBHC process is based on real clinical decisions, focuses on learners' actual learning needs, and connects what is already known by the student with the new knowledge. It is also important that the teacher makes explicit how to appraise the evidence and apply it to a patient's care in an integrated manner, thus seamlessly incorporating EBHC into the clinical experience. This latter concept has been the guiding principle in attempts to restructure the clinical curriculum.

However, they also discuss some of the mistakes they have made (**Box 1**), which include emphasizing how to "do" research over how to "use" research findings. EBHC should also be seen as a method to not only find flaws in the published literature but also identify evidence that can provide therapeutic guidance. If EBHC sessions

---

Box 1
Mistakes to avoid in teaching evidence-based health care

1. Emphasize how to do research rather than how to use research findings to inform clinical practice

2. Emphasize how to perform statistical analyses rather than how to interpret the results of such analyses

3. Find only flaws in the published literature, rather than also trying to find information that offers clinical guidance

4. Cast EBHC as a substitute for the clinician's judgment and skills rather than as a complement to them

5. Disconnect the EBHC process from the clinical process and the team's need for clinical information

6. Exceed the amount of time available and/or the teams' attention span

7. Humiliate the learner for not knowing some bit of clinical information

8. Strive for full educational closure by the end of the session, rather than leaving some aspects unresolved to encourage the student to think and learn between sessions

become exercises in which no evidence is seen as valid, the result is a "therapeutic nihilism" in which the teacher is reluctant to recommend any treatment. Evidence-based care often provides a bias toward rational action, not therapeutic nihilism. [29,30] Students must learn not only to critique the literature for errors but also obtain useful information that may be used in caring for their patients.

One other mistake is the assumption that learning occurs only during formal course sessions. Clinical learning should occur in the context of patient care, which is why the authors have chosen to attempt to fully integrate EBHC within their clinical teaching and patient care missions. Only then will students see EBHC for what it is: a practical tool for clinical practice, rather than a sterile academic exercise.

THE GRADUATE PERIODONTOLOGY EXPERIENCE

The first academic unit of the University of Kentucky to implement a comprehensive evidence-based curriculum was the Graduate Periodontology Program (GPP). Consequently, most of the authors' experience has been in this program. In 2000, work was begun on a set of clinical protocols that were developed according to the principles of evidence-based medicine (**Table 1**). Whenever possible, systematic reviews and meta-analyses were used, but when these were unavailable, primary literature searches were undertaken. Studies with multiple research hypotheses, small sample sizes, and other deficiencies were not assigned the same importance as systematic reviews and meta-analyses. These protocols were collected into a manual, which is provided in both hard-copy and online formats.[31] The contents of the manual have been used to inform teaching, research, and service in the program. When insufficient high-quality evidence existed, the choices became more difficult.

Teaching

The clinical protocols and the reviews on which they are based form the foundation for most of the didactic education in the GPP. The diagnostic and clinical protocols are periodically reviewed in one of the graduate seminars. A rotating series of topics (each corresponding to a diagnostic or treatment protocol) is covered over the course of a 2-year cycle. All residents participate in this seminar. Before the seminar, one resident is assigned the role of moderator and reviews the evidence regarding the topic. Systematic reviews and meta-analyses are used whenever available. The moderator appraises the evidence and then presents the findings to the group during the actual seminar session. If the evidence supports the protocol, it is simply reviewed and an updated (but essentially unchanged) protocol is filed in the program manual (which is available online and in hard-copy format). If new evidence has sufficient strength, then the protocol may be modified or amended and the protocol entry in the program manual changed accordingly (see **Table 1**).

In extreme cases, a protocol could be rejected or superseded by another procedure. Residents and faculty can suggest new interventions that may also be reviewed in the format of this seminar. In this way, the protocols are continuously reviewed and updated, graduate students develop strong expertise in and appreciation of EBHC methodology, and patient care is based on the best available evidence. Plans are underway to make this library available to alumni of the program and other interested parties.

To further integrating evidence and clinical education, the basic science curriculum is coordinated so that basic biomedical science and related clinical topics are covered together (to the extent possible). For example, certain aspects of bone biology are covered during the same period that literature reviews on regenerative therapy are

Table 1
Clinical protocol based on principles of evidence-based medicine

Parameter	Details
Condition	Chronic periodontitis of early-advanced severity
Patient	Any
Intervention[a]	Initial therapy (to consist of SRP/subgingival debridement, oral hygiene assessment and instruction, smoking cessation (if appropriate), extraction of hopeless teeth (see appropriate protocol – or these might be listed here [eg, class III mobility/depressible, radiographic bone loss > 75%]) Initial therapy must always be followed by a formal reevaluation (ie, comprehensive periodontal examination) 4 to 8 weeks following last session of scaling and root planning (SRP) As an alternative to conventional SRP, a full-mouth debridement can be carried out in two appointments over 24 to 48 hours
Compared with	Conventional initial therapy vs. full-mouth debridement vs. coronal scaling and polishing
Outcome	Initial therapy effective, although coronal scaling and polishing is not (in terms of improving surrogate indices). In patients with chronic periodontitis in moderately deep pockets slightly more favorable outcomes for pocket reduction and gain in probing attachment were found following FMD compared with control.
Recommendation	Diagnosis of chronic periodontitis requires initial therapy. FMD may provide a slight additional benefit in some cases
Sources	Eberhard J, Jepsen S, Jervøe-Storm PM, et al. Full-mouth disinfection for the treatment of adult chronic periodontitis. Cochrane Database Syst Rev 2008;(1):CD004622; and
	Hung HC, Douglass CW. Meta-analysis of the effect of scaling and root planing, surgical treatment and antibiotic therapies on periodontal probing depth and attachment loss. J Clin Periodontol 2002;29(11): 975–86.
Strength of evidence	High
Review date	September 2008
Author(s)	M. V. Thomas

[a] The treatment protocol presumes that thorough initial examination and risk-assessment was completed, including medical consultation and clearance as needed.

being conducted. This coordination results in a synergistic learning experience in which clinical intervention and basic biomedical science are coupled in a rational way.

Research

EBHC also has a significant impact on clinical research. One obvious example is the requirement to track and report clinical outcomes and adverse events. For example, the authors implemented a quality assurance initiative designed to assess patient-centered outcomes in their implant program from 2000 to 2008.

EBHC can also enhance research efforts through identifying gaps in knowledge. An example is that of the palatal implant anchorage system. Several years ago, a small implant was developed to provide anchorage to enhance orthodontic tooth movement.[32] This implant was designed to be placed in the midline of the palate. Few studies had been reported on the palatal implant at that time, because it was only recently developed. Having performed a few mock procedures on cadavers, the authors were concerned about the possibility of inadvertently perforating the nasal cavity during implant placement. To evaluate the risk of this surgical misadventure, the authors reviewed the literature regarding thickness of the maxillary palate and concluded that information regarding the thickness of the bony palate was insufficient to allow an evidence-based risk estimate. As a result of this dearth of evidence, a series of cadaver studies were conducted to assess the mean palatal thickness and likelihood of nasal perforation subsequent to implant placement.[32–34]

These studies determined that the floor of the nasal cavity could be perforated during placement of the palatal implants, but that this hazard could be radically reduced when using the shorter (ie, 4 mm) implant and placing it in a paramedian location.[33] Thus, although not performing a randomized controlled trial designed to compare interventions, the authors were nonetheless able to suggest a possible source of patient harm and suggest steps that could be taken to reduce this risk. Risk reduction and optimization of patient outcomes are at the core of the EBHC concept. This example also shows that lower levels of evidence may occasionally be informative and useful in guiding clinical decision-making.

Service

Experts hope that adopting specific evidence-based protocols will improve consistency of services and have a positive effect on patient outcomes. Although this assumption is plausible, it must be tested. The use of these protocols should also help provide consistency and calibration of the various full- and part-time attending faculty members. This calibration, however, has proven to be somewhat more challenging than the authors initially believed, partly because of difficulties in communicating effectively with all part- and full-time faculty. The authors are currently creating research protocols to quantify the effect of EBHC on both patient outcomes and provider consistency.

Program Evaluation

The final step in teaching EBHC is self-evaluation. In this regard, Straus and colleagues[11] suggest several questions that must be answered. Following are questions and corresponding answers as applied to the authors' EBHC-based curriculum in GPP.

Am I Asking Any Clinical Questions at All?

After several years, this is being done regularly basis by the graduate students, the program director, and some of the faculty. Asking clinical questions is so much a part of the program that it does not seem to be a separate and distinct exercise. Recently, a resident was presented with a clinical situation involving a crown–implant ratio exceeding 1:1. A prosthodontic faculty member informed the resident that this ratio could not exceed 1:1 or implant failure would likely result. The resident was unwilling to accept this on the faculty member's authority alone (ie, in the absence of valid evidence), and found a 10-year prospective study that addressed this question. The authors reported that "implant restorations with C/I ratios between 2 and 3 may be successfully used in the posterior areas of the jaw."[35] As a result of experiencing almost 3 years of an evidence-based curriculum, the student instinctively responded to this question by conducting a focused literature search, retrieving a relevant study, and ranking that study according to the hierarchy of evidence (as relatively weak, but suggestive, evidence).

Am I Asking Well-Formulated Questions?

Most questions asked in the GPP were formulated in roughly the same format as described by Straus and colleagues[11] for both background and foreground questions.

Are We Saving the Questions (and Answers) in Some Readily Accessible Database?

It is critical to the success of the project that the results of searches be maintained in a readily accessible (and searchable) repository. There have been some frustrations, but an online SharePoint site is now being used with reasonable success. The college is currently implementing a similar predoctoral EBHC initiative (described later). The predoctoral initiative consists of a series of discipline-specific clinical protocols that will be accessible at the point-of-care in online and hard-copy formats.

PREDOCTORAL CURRICULUM

The success of EBHC-based curricula in GPP suggested that a similar approach might be tried in the predoctoral clinical curriculum. An evidence-based curriculum enhancement project was undertaken that is similar in concept to that used in Graduate Periodontology.

Meetings were held with the division chiefs of the selected clinical disciplines. They were given an overview of the EBHC process and some examples of clinical decision-making tools.[36] The divisions were charged with developing diagnostic and treatment protocols for the most common procedures performed in their discipline. These protocols were to be based on best evidence and developed over 9-months. These protocols are designed to facilitate clinical decision-making at the point-of-care, and include several clinical decision support tools, some of which are available through the ADA.[36]

The proposal has had a surprising amount of support from most disciplines. Protocols are currently being received and posted to the online site, after vetting by a committee overseeing the process. The project will be monitored for effectiveness over the next 12 months, including degree of compliance with posted protocols, attitudes of the various stakeholders (faculty, staff, and students), and selected patient outcomes. These data will be used to improve and refine the program. The authors hope to create a self-sustaining database that can be used to inform patient care and clinical education, while providing students with a model for rational, evidence-based practice. Readers who are interested in accessing the site should contact the corresponding author.

CHALLENGES IN IMPLEMENTING AN EVIDENCE-BASED CURRICULUM

Several hurdles must be overcome in implementing an evidence-based foundation in either practice or academic healthcare. One challenge is inherent in the biomedical literature; evidence is insufficient to support or refute many interventions. Some of this is because of flaws in trial design, as reported by Hujoel.[37] In some cases, no trials have been conducted. In either event, one may have little or no "best evidence" on which to make a decision. This enigma is discussed at length in the paper by Bader elsewhere in this issue. Matthews[38] recently presented a practical approach to this problem in which best evidence is sought and appraised, consistent with EBHC practice. If the evidence is insufficient to provide clear guidance, then clinicians must use the best evidence available and develops a "script" in which the degree of uncertainty is presented to the patient, along with the options for treatment. In his brief description of this process, he cites some clinical examples, including what to tell a pregnant patient who has periodontitis who is concerned about the possibility of miscarriage:

Mrs. M, our examination reveals you have moderate periodontal disease. This means you have inflamed gums and some loss of attachment between the gums and teeth. I have conducted a thorough search of the best scientific evidence. This shows a weak association between periodontal disease and adverse pregnancy outcomes, but does now show that periodontitis causes miscarriage. We do not have enough data to say with certainty that periodontal disease causes health problems in the newborn. There is evidence that nonsurgical periodontal treatment is safe during pregnancy, however. Without treatment, your gum disease may become worse, which will likely result in loss of bone and, perhaps, teeth. Some studies who improved pregnancy outcomes after periodontal treatment, but some do not. There is no evidence that such treatment is harmful to the unborn child.

This scripted answer to the patient's query is an accurate reflection of the current (and somewhat ambiguous) state of the research literature.[39–42]

Another challenge in implementing EBHC is the resistance to change by clinicians. When introduced to the concept of EBHC, some respond by asking "Isn't this what we have always done?" This is a reasonable question. To some extent, physicians and dentists have based their treatment decisions on research findings. However, the emphasis on ranking the evidence, heavy reliance on the systematic review and meta-analysis, and emphasis on collecting and organizing the results of evidence appraisals make EBHC sufficiently different as to warrant its status as a concept that differs from what was previously done. This distinction is particularly true in light of literature that suggests that physicians and dentists often do not provide care that is consistent with the best evidence.

One mundane, but troublesome, problem the authors encountered was a lack of time on the part of the faculty. Because of time constraints the pace of generating protocols has been slower than desired. To overcome this inertia, having one of the EBD champions meet with groups of clinicians to help develop questions to be answered was found to be helpful. This process was sometimes effective in providing the impetus to stimulate more activity. In addition, providing students with the experience of assisting with the evidence-gathering process (under the guidance of faculty experienced in EBHC) had the dual advantage of teaching EBHC in a hands-on setting and providing help to time-constrained faculty.

Another practical problem is disseminating the EBHC process (and, later, protocols) to all faculty, including those who teach on a part-time basis. For two consecutive years at Kentucky, a portion of the annual faculty retreats was used to disseminate information on the basic EBHC process and methodology before the rollout of the predoctoral EBHC initiative. This technique may have made the concepts more familiar and less threatening to the faculty, although that assumption has not been tested.

EBHC may be threatening to some clinicians who might fear loss of autonomy and that EBHC will be used by third-party payers to dictate treatment and thereby have a potential adverse effect practitioner income. These concerns are really separate. Regarding a loss of autonomy, the EBHC process calls for "the integration of the best research evidence with our clinical expertise and our patient's unique values and circumstances."[11] Note that best evidence must always be applied in the light of the clinician's knowledge and experience, and that the needs and preferences of the individual patient are paramount. EBHC is not "cookbook medicine" but rather a rational method of approaching clinical problems.

Regarding third-party payers, it is possible that they might use EBHC concepts to dictate treatment or restrict choices on economic grounds (to the detriment of the practitioner). However, the opposite may also be true. If, for example, "best evidence" shows that periodontal treatment reduces the risk for preterm birth, medical insurance carriers may choose to cover these interventions. In any event, practitioners should base their decisions or recommendations on sound evidence.

Lastly, clinical recommendations can be no better than the decisions on which they are based. If the authors of a systematic review allow their biases to influence the selection of manuscripts to be reviewed or some other aspect of the analysis, the evidence will be tainted and may be invalid. For this reason, editors of biomedical journals must overcome the aversion to publish confirmatory investigations and reviews; it is often valuable when two or more groups publish systematic reviews on the same topic and reach the same conclusions. When only one review is available, readers should use caution in applying the results.

In summary, implementing EBHC in the academic dental setting has several challenges. However, once the process is underway, it ceases to be seen as something different from and external to the clinical decision-making process. The goal at Kentucky is to achieve the goal of weaving the evidence into clinical and didactic efforts so thoroughly and seamlessly that it is invisible to students and faculty. This attitude regarding the use of evidence can eventually become second-nature, so that practitioners are not conscious of practicing EBHC.

SUMMARY

UKCD has chosen to base its curriculum and clinical care on an evidence-based model. Students must become both "users" and "doers" of EBHC, but the emphasis is clearly on "doing." The authors believe that integrating EBHC into the clinical and didactic curriculum will yield significant advantages because students will learn the tools of EBHC through actually applying these principles to treatment, and then carry these tools into practice.

REFERENCES

1. Sackett DL, Rosenberg WM, Gray JA, et al. Evidence based medicine: what it is and what it isn't. BMJ 1996;312(7023):71–2.
2. Hujoel P. Grading the evidence: the core of EBD. J Evid Based Dent Pract 2008; 8(3):116–8.
3. Sackett D, Haynes R, Tugwell P, et al. Clinical epidemiology: a basic science for clinical medicine. Philadelphia: Lippincott Williams and Wilkins; 1991. p. 441.
4. Porter ME, Teisberg EO. Redefining health care: creating value-based competition on results. Boston: Harvard Business School Press; 2006.
5. Mangione-Smith R, DeCristofaro AH, Setodji CM, et al. The quality of ambulatory care delivered to children in the United States. N Engl J Med 2007;357(15): 1515–23.
6. McGlynn EA, Asch SM, Adams J, et al. The quality of health care delivered to adults in the United States. N Engl J Med 2003;348(26):2635–45.

7. Garvin J. In: ADA brings evidence-based dentistry to the grassroots. vol. 2008. American Dental Association; 2008.

8. Frantsve-Hawley J, Meyer DM. The evidence-based dentistry champions: a grassroots approach to the implementation of EBD. J Evid Based Dent Pract 2008;8(2):64–9.

9. Frantsve-Hawley J, Newman MG, Meyer DM. Proceedings of the evidence-based dentistry champion conference. Introduction. J Evid Based Dent Pract 2008;8(3): 113–4.

10. Newman MG, Frantsve-Hawley J, Meyer DM. 3rd International conference on evidence-based dentistry. Introduction. J Evid Based Dent Pract 2008;8(3):162.

11. Straus SE, Richardon WS, Glasziou P, et al. Evidence-based medicine: how to practice and teach EBM. Edinburgh: Elsevier Churchill Livingstone; 2005.

12. Mark DB. Decision-making in clinical medicine. In: Kasper DL, Braunwald E, Fauci AS, editors. Harrison's principles of internal medicine. New York: McGraw-Hill; 2005. p. 6–12.

13. Galanter WL, Hier DB, Jao C, et al. Computerized physician order entry of medications and clinical decision support can improve problem list documentation compliance. Int J Med Inf 2008.

14. Kuperman GJ, Bobb A, Payne TH, et al. Medication-related clinical decision support in computerized provider order entry systems: a review. J Am Med Inform Assoc 2007;14(1):29–40.

15. Last JM. A Dictionary of epidemiology. Oxford: Oxford University Press; 2001.

16. Chiller KG, Washington C, Sober AJ, et al. Cancer of the skin. In: Kasper DL, Braunwald E, Fauci AS, editors. Harrison's principles of internal medicine. New York: McGraw-Hill; 2005. p. 497–503.

17. Lopez NJ, Jara L, Valenzuela CY. Association of interleukin-1 polymorphisms with periodontal disease. J Periodontol 2005;76(2):234–43.

18. Quappe L, Jara L, Lopez NJ. Association of interleukin-1 polymorphisms with aggressive periodontitis. J Periodontol 2004;75(11):1509–15.

19. Kornman KS, Crane A, Wang HY, et al. The interleukin-1 genotype as a severity factor in adult periodontal disease. J Clin Periodontol 1997;24(1):72–7.

20. Armitage GC, Wu Y, Wang HY, et al. Low prevalence of a periodontitis-associated interleukin-1 composite genotype in individuals of Chinese heritage. J Periodontol 2000;71(2):164–71.

21. Azarpazhooh A, Mayhall JT, Leake JL. Introducing dental students to evidence-based decisions in dental care. J Dent Educ 2008;72(1):87–109.

22. Faggion CM Jr, Tu YK. Evidence-based dentistry: a model for clinical practice. J Dent Educ 2007;71(6):825–31.

23. Levine AE, Bebermeyer RD, Chen JW, et al. Development of an interdisciplinary course in information resources and evidence-based dentistry. J Dent Educ 2008;72(9):1067–76.

24. Sackett DL, Straus SE. Finding and applying evidence during clinical rounds: the "evidence cart". J Am Med Assoc 1998;280(15):1336–8.

25. Frantsve-Hawley J. Evidence locator: sources of evidence-based dentistry information. J Evid Based Dent Pract 2008;8(3):133–8.

26. Richards D, Clarkson J, Matthews D, et al. Evidence-based dentistry: managing information for better practice. London: Quintessence; 2008.

27. Korenstein D, Dunn A, McGinn T. Mixing it up: integrating evidence-based medicine and patient care. Acad Med 2002;77(7):741–2.

28. Sackett D, Strauss S, Richardson W, et al. Evidence-based medicine: how to practice and teach EBM. Edinburgh: Churchill Livingstone; 2000.

29. Fillit HM, Doody RS, Binaso K, et al. Recommendations for best practices in the treatment of Alzheimer's disease in managed care. Am J Geriatr Pharmacother 2006;4(Suppl A):S9–24 [quiz S25–8].
30. Heinz A, Wilwer M, Mann K. Therapy and supportive care of alcoholics: guidelines for practitioners. Best Pract Res Clin Gastroenterol 2003;17(4):695–708.
31. Thomas MV. A clinical mariner's guide to the uncharted sea of patient care: the university of Kentucky graduate periodontology program manual. Lexington (KY): University of Kentucky; 2007.
32. Thomas MV, Daniel TL, Kluemper T. Implant anchorage in orthodontic practice: the Straumann orthosystem. Dent Clin North Am 2006;50(3):425–37.
33. Daniel TL. Nasal perforation secondary to paramedian palatal orthodontic implant placement. Lexington (KY): University of Kentucky; 2005. p. 30.
34. Dyer CE. Median and paramedian palatal bone thickness available for orthodontic implant placement: a cadaver study. Lexington (KY): University of Kentucky; 2005. p. 36.
35. Blanes RJ, Bernard JP, Blanes ZM, et al. A 10-year prospective study of ITI dental implants placed in the posterior region. II: influence of the crown-to-implant ratio and different prosthetic treatment modalities on crestal bone loss. Clin Oral Implants Res 2007;18(6):707–14.
36. Merijohn GK, Bader JD, Frantsve-Hawley J, et al. Clinical decision support chairside tools for evidence-based dental practice. J Evid Based Dent Pract 2008; 8(3):119–32.
37. Hujoel PP. Definitive vs exploratory periodontal trials: a survey of published studies. J Dent Res 1995;74(8):1453–8.
38. Matthews J. Emerging issues in dentistry: caring for patients in the absence of evidence. J Evid Based Dent Pract 2008;8(3):139–43.
39. Michalowicz BS, Hodges JS, DiAngelis AJ, et al. Treatment of periodontal disease and the risk of preterm birth. N Engl J Med 2006;355(18):1885–94.
40. Offenbacher S, Lin D, Strauss R, et al. Effects of periodontal therapy during pregnancy on periodontal status, biologic parameters, and pregnancy outcomes: a pilot study. J Periodontol 2006;77(12):2011–24.
41. Vergnes JN. Studies suggest an association between maternal periodontal disease and pre-eclampsia. Evid Based Dent 2008;9(2):46–7.
42. Vergnes JN, Sixou M. Preterm low birth weight and maternal periodontal status: a meta-analysis. Am J Obstet Gynecol 2007;196(2):135, e1–7.

Stumbling into the Age of Evidence

James D. Bader, DDS, MPH

KEYWORDS

- Evidence-based dentistry • Dental knowledgebase
- Systematic reviews

This article presents personal observations on how the concept of evidence-based dentistry is faring in the profession. It considers how the dental profession's concept of evidence has matured, how evidence-based dentistry was originally envisioned, how it is currently embodied, and what its prospects might be for the immediate future.

Evidence-based dentistry began in the profession approximately 2 decades ago, initiated by the appearance of the first systematic reviews on dental topics in the late 1980s.[1] The emergence of the concept of evidence-based dentistry—and its fundamental construct, the systematic review—marks what can be considered a fundamental shift in how the dental knowledge base has grown and developed over time.

EVOLUTION OF THE DENTAL KNOWLEDGE BASE

The dental knowledge base defines the profession of dentistry and influences how dentists practice. It is a store of special information about oral health and diseases, treatment methods, and their outcomes. It serves as the basis for professional decision making, and portions of it form the principal content of predoctoral and postdoctoral dental curricula. The knowledge base has evolved in how knowledge has been created, synthesized, and disseminated. Four eras, or ages, can be delineated in the evolution of the knowledge base (**Table 1**), and a brief consideration of these ages may help put the profession's current involvement in evidence-based dentistry into perspective.

The dental knowledge base first began to develop during the "Age of the Expert." Dentistry emerged in the middle ages as a guild of "barber surgeons" and "itinerant dentists." Knowledge creation was strictly experiential, and little systematized observation was available. Knowledge synthesis was little more than deepening experience, with virtually no texts and limited opportunities for sharing knowledge among practitioners who were mostly illiterate and restricted in travel radius. Similarly, knowledge dissemination was restricted, informal, and limited principally to the master–apprentice relationship, wherein *experts* passed on their synthesis of experience to one or more novices.

Operative Dentistry CB# 7450, School of Dentistry, University of North Carolina, Chapel Hill, NC 27599, USA
E-mail address: jim_bader@unc.edu

Dent Clin N Am 53 (2009) 15–22
doi:10.1016/j.cden.2008.09.001
0011-8532/08/$ – see front matter © 2009 Elsevier Inc. All rights reserved.

Table 1 Evolution of the dental knowledge base			
	Principal Method for Knowledge Base Process		
Era	**Knowledge Creation**	**Knowledge Synthesis**	**Knowledge Dissemination**
Age of the Expert	Experiential	Experimental	Apprenticeship
Age of Professionalization	Experiential limited observational	Shared experimental	Texts, societies, journals, schools
Age of Science	Experiential	Traditional literature review	Texts, journals, schools, formal CE
Age of Evidence	Experiential	Systematic review	Texts, journals, schools, CE, guidelines, evidence summaries

Around the middle of the 18th century, the dental knowledge base entered the second era, the "Age of Professionalization." Fauchard had published his comprehensive textbook, representing his observations, those of his mentor, other dentists at the hospital where he practiced, and, later, other experts in Paris. This better access to knowledge created by others led to a greater degree of knowledge synthesis, exemplified by Fauchard's text and others. However, what was synthesized was still simply the experience of others.

Available texts initially represented the most important improvement in dissemination of the knowledge base, with later improvements accruing through the establishment of dental schools and the first dental society journals in the 1840s. The age of professionalization also saw the some growth of controlled experimentation for the creation of new knowledge, again focused primarily on treatment of dental disease.

The dental knowledge base entered the third era, the "Age of Science," at approximately the dawn of the 20th century, presaging the profession's gradual shift from proprietary educational to university-based institutions. Knowledge creation accelerated as protocol-based experimentation became more common, and the scope of inquiry broadened to more fully include the causes and prevention of disease.

Knowledge synthesis evolved slowly, from simple statements of fact based on an expert's experience, toward consideration of the available knowledge in scientific literature. The product of this evolution was the traditional review of literature, with the expert remaining the key element of the review, selecting the studies to be included and providing a subjective interpretation of this literature. Thus, the synthesis was open to bias, both intended and unintentional. This phase marked the most active period of knowledge dissemination, with early rapid growth of university-based pre- and postdoctoral dental curricula and both early and more recent proliferations of journals, and organized continuing dental education in journals.

It can be argued that the dental knowledge base is now entering a fourth era: the "Age of Evidence." Knowledge creation in this era can be characterized by the dominance of randomized clinical trials, although observational study designs continue to be used, with valuable information contributed through improved multivariate statistical methods.

A change in the principal method of knowledge synthesis represents the hallmark of the Age of Evidence, with the traditional literature review superseded by the systematic review. Systematic reviews represent a substantial change in the paradigm of synthesis through ensuring inclusion of all relevant evidence, deemphasizing the role of the expert, and minimizing bias through strict protocols demanding objectivity and transparency in the review process.

Systematic reviews have been published with ever-increasing frequency in the past decade,[1] and probably now number more than 700. The methods of knowledge dissemination dominant in the previous era (eg, dental curricula, texts, scientific journals, continuing dental education) continue to be prominent, but initial signs of change also are apparent. Two distillations of the results of systematic reviews are growing more evident within the profession. Evidence-based clinical guidelines promulgated by various agencies and societies are increasingly common, and evidence summaries—essentially abstracts of systematic reviews accompanied by critical commentaries—form most of the content of two dental journals,[2,3] and appear occasionally in others.

Perhaps the most significant change in the dissemination of the dental knowledge base in these early years of the Age of Evidence is easy access to the substantial majority of the knowledge base through the Internet. For the first time, the general public can, with little special effort, access the information that theoretically drives dentists' diagnostic and treatment decisions. The ramifications of this open access to the core of the profession have yet to fully manifest. Patient consultations that include a debate of the merits of the exclusion criteria of a newly released systematic review may not yet be possible, but expecting at least some patients to be aware of their diagnoses, reasonably well informed, and prepared to discuss their treatment options may be realistic.

EVIDENCE-BASED DENTISTRY AS INITIALLY ENVISIONED

When the concept of evidence-based health care first began to gain momentum in the health sciences in the late 1980s and early 1990s, the general assumption was that individual clinicians would become experts in interpreting the original scientific literature and applying the fruits of that appraisal to their practices. *The Journal of the American Medical Association (JAMA)* ran a lengthy series of Users' Guides to the Medical Literature developed by the Evidence-Based Working Group.[4,5] In the words of the Working Group:

> Clinicians need to be able to distinguish high from low quality in primary studies, systematic reviews, practice guidelines, and other integrative research focused management recommendations. An evidence-based practitioner must also understand the patient's circumstances or predicament; identify knowledge gaps and frame questions to fill those gaps; critically appraise the research evidence and apply that evidence to patient care.[6]

To assist in these endeavors, attention was paid to making the literature accessible to clinicians at the bedside.[7]

The expectations in dentistry were similar. British dentists practicing evidence-based dentistry were envisioned as identifying the evidence online, critically appraising it, and acting on it.[8] However, an early note of caution was expressed regarding dentists' abilities to marshal the thought processes necessary for these tasks, although the problem was seen as being overcome to some extent by the development of computer programs teaching probabilistic thinking.[9] The principal outcome associated with adopting evidence-based dentistry was to have better information, which was assumed to translate to a more knowledgeable practitioner.[8-10] At the same time, evidence-based dentistry was seen as informing dental researchers and educators, thereby improving their insight and methods.[11] Downstream benefits were expected to include more effective treatment and cost savings.[8]

Early in the development of the evidence-based care movement in all health disciplines, the actual knowledge translation process was given little attention. The belief seemed to be widely held that the availability of more accurate information would lead to its uptake by most practitioners, leading to behavioral change. Furthermore, evidence-based practice guidelines were envisioned to be a substantial mechanism for change, with widespread adherence seemingly taken for granted. The overriding issue that evidence-based care could address was a lack of focused information addressing clinical problems, and thus the unwarranted reliance on experts or authorities.[8] The availability and quality of evidence that addressed the problems of clinical practice were not often mentioned as a concern, and when availability was addressed it was seen as a limited problem.[9]

Thus, it is not overreaching to conclude that, in the early flush of excitement over the development and implementation of evidence-based care concepts, a somewhat optimistic and uncritical attitude prevailed in the health care professions regarding the promise that these concepts held for patients and the health professions. In retrospect, it is somewhat surprising that this attitude could have flourished, because it was already well established that attempts to translate research findings into practice through conventional means were neither efficient nor effective.[11,12]

EVIDENCE-BASED DENTISTRY IN REALITY

Almost 2 decades into the putative age of evidence in the dental profession, the assumptions that have borne little fruit are easy to identify. The greatest disappointments have been that most clinicians have not become discriminating consumers of the research literature, that the promised answers to clinical dilemmas have not always emerged from the evidence, and that dentists still misinterpret the principles and purposes of evidence-based dentistry.

Although current assessments of dentists' sources of information are lacking, indirect evidence suggests that dentists seldom read and evaluate the original research literature.[13,14] Rather, they read summaries in their professional journals and continue to rely on other sources of information, most notably their colleagues and continuing education presentations.[15,16] Chairside computing is available to few dentists,[17] limiting opportunities to conduct real-time patient-specific searches. This disappointment really should not be regarded as unexpected. The assumption that dentists would find time and resources to add searching, reading, and assessing the literature to an already long list of activities and responsibilities crowding their daily schedule was probably both impractical and unrealistic.

In reality, evidence-based dentistry has not brought a great wave of needed clinical answers to the profession. To illustrate that contention, consider the findings of the 80 published Cochrane reviews.[18] Of these reviews, 35 (44%) could not answer the clinical question they set out to address because of insufficient evidence. Another 32 (40%) answered the question, with 22 finding the intervention in question to be effective and 10 finding no difference among the interventions in question. Finally, the answers to the 13 remaining questions (16%) were "hedged" because of weak evidence or lack of clinical significance. Thus, an unequivocal answer was produced for few questions. This disappointing result also could have been anticipated,[9] which might have mitigated current negative attitudes toward evidence-based dentistry. Because evidence-based dentistry had been touted early as a means of answering vexing clinical questions, the frequent absence of definitive answers is understandably frustrating to clinicians.

Furthering that frustration is the fact that some unanswered questions address controversial issues for which the profession would be expected to cite substantial available supporting evidence, given its avowed policies. For example, "conventional wisdom" among dentists has long held that patients should be seen at least every 6 months, and that dental examinations should be accompanied by scaling and polishing. However, systematic reviews could not show convincing evidence of the necessity of semiannual application of either procedure.[19,20]

A final concern is voiced principally by academics: although a large number of systematic reviews is now available in the literature,[1] not all reviews have been performed at a level that meets recommended standards.[21] Thus, some reviews may reflect bias, the bane of the traditional literature review that systematic reviews are designed to minimize.

Misconceptions about evidence-based dentistry are frequent among clinicians. To some, citing a single study as the evidence supporting a treatment decision is synonymous with practicing evidence-based dentistry. What is not appreciated is that *evidence* means all the evidence, as assembled and assessed through a systematic review. Others still believe that evidence-based dentistry is an unwarranted intrusion into practice, in essence telling a clinician what to do. However, what is not appreciated is that evidence-based dentistry simply provides a clinician with complete, unbiased information about alternative treatments or a prognosis for a clinical condition. Clinicians must recommend treatment for a given patient by integrating the evidence-based information on treatment effectiveness or prognosis with their assessment of the patient, including the clinical condition of interest, comorbidities, and risk factors.

Despite the disappointments, frustrations, and misconceptions, the profession is accommodating to evidence-based dentistry and is benefiting from some of its early outcomes. For example, systematic reviews have helped resolve some clinical issues, such as the relative effectiveness of endodontic treatment and implant therapy,[22,23] while challenging entrenched conventional wisdom surrounding other issues.[19,20] As another example, a recent assessment of the evidence indicated that rather than not using sealants because of concern about "sealing in" caries, clinicians should consider dental sealants an effective treatment for occlusal enamel caries.[24,25] Furthermore, the need for evidence, so obviously shown in systematic reviews that failed to answer common clinical questions, was an important factor in the decision by the National Institute for Dental and Carniofacial Research to support three practice-based research networks that are now in their third year of operation, and to add research findings to the evidence base.[26–28] Dental school curricula are being revised to include basic information on evidence-based dentistry concepts and evidence-based dental practice, and to ensure that course content is evidence-based.[29,30] Currently, two dental journals are available whose contents are devoted almost entirely to evidence-based dentistry.[2,3] All of these developments indicate a increasing emphasis on evidence from the dental knowledge base for guiding clinical practice.

Despite these positive signs, there are currently no firm indications of an "evidence-based dentistry effect" on clinician behavior and, ultimately, patient outcomes. One might conjecture that evidence-based dentistry's real value has been to remind clinicians that their daily treatment decisions should be based on the evidence, when available, and, by implication, that they should be amenable to changing those decisions when evidence becomes available suggesting that an alternative treatment would provide greater benefit to their patients. In fact, there are some suggestions that even this hoped-for effect is less than pervasive. The few evaluations of clinicians' adherence to evidence-based treatment guidelines indicate only limited compliance, despite attempts to communicate the evidence-based nature of the treatment recommendations.[31–33]

WHERE EVIDENCE-BASED DENTISTRY IS GOING

Despite the profession's initial lukewarm embrace of evidence-based dentistry, there are no signs that the concept will be abandoned. Systematic reviews, which are the cornerstone of evidence-based dentistry, continue to appear, seemingly at an accelerating rate. Dental schools continue to validate evidence-based dentistry through exemplifying and teaching its precepts in their curricula. These two processes—synthesizing the evidence and preparing the next generation of dentists to anticipate, seek, and welcome new information and modify their clinical behavior accordingly—virtually guarantee that evidence-based dental practice will flourish in the long-term. The real question is what will happen in the next few years in the arena of dental practice.

Despite Yogi Berra's warning that "it's tough to make predictions, especially about the future,"[34] it is fairly easy to forecast that evidence-based dentistry will increasingly influence the practice of dentistry, although the road will be bumpy in the near future. Progress will come largely from the emphasis that the American Dental Association (ADA) is placing on evidence-based dentistry. The ADA is overhauling its Web site, which will be designed to provide "one-stop" evidence-based dentistry services, including an up-to-date indexed listing of all published systematic reviews on clinical dental topics, commentaries on selected reviews, and links to other review summaries and clinical recommendations.[35] The ADA is also organizing a 3-year program to encourage the adoption of evidence-based dental practice among clinicians. After training workshops, "evidence-based dentistry champions" will seek opportunities to disseminate information about evidence-based dentistry to their colleagues.[36]

The bumps in the road will come from two sources. The primary source is clinical inertia: dentists are slow to change, despite knowing that change is indicated.[37] The problem is ubiquitous in the health professions and effective solutions have been slow to materialize. Provision of knowledge usually is not enough to overcome inertia. More complex, coordinated interventions are necessary, and these are difficult in the relatively isolated environment of dental practice. Evidence-based dental practice requires change in clinical behaviors, and until dentists can be induced to change when the evidence suggests that they should, progress toward evidence-based care will inevitably suffer.

The other impediment to change is a combination of fear and suspicion. Most dentists are businesspersons, and are therefore sensitive to threats to their revenue steam. Evidence-based dentistry can be seen as both a legitimate and an illegitimate threat to that stream. Legitimate threats arise when the evidence suggests that patients benefit less from or pay more for a given treatment or clinical protocol than an alternative that is financially less rewarding to the dental practice. Fortunately, these circumstances are becoming less frequent as dentistry continues to phase out surgical approaches to treatment held over from a time of elevated caries and periodontal disease incidence. Illegitimate threats can occur when carriers cite evidence as the basis for policy decisions regarding reimbursement for certain procedures, and the evidence is something other than the results of a systematic review. Carriers may have the right to set reimbursement policy, but citing their own claims experience as the "evidence" supporting the policy represents regression to an earlier age in the dental knowledge base, and inevitably casts evidence-based dentistry in a bad light.

Therefore, the near-term future for evidence-based dental practice is likely to be characterized by continuation of current trends in dissemination of evidence-based information to clinicians. The primary means for that dissemination will consist of evidence summaries and evidence-based treatment recommendations and guidelines. Evidence summaries are a rapid, accessible means of presenting the results and clinical implications of a systematic review, and they are beginning to appear in various journals and other formats. Evidence-based treatment guidelines are also appearing with greater frequency, promulgated by a wide variety of voluntary organizations. Although neither of these means of dissemination will be markedly more effective in changing clinicians' behavior than more traditional information dissemination methods, they will ensure that the knowledge is evidence-based. This process, in itself, is an important, albeit preliminary step in ensuring that the profession provides evidence-based care to its patients.

REFERENCES

1. Bader J, Ismail A. Survey of systematic reviews in dentistry. J Am Dent Assoc 2004;135:464–73.
2. Evidence-based dentistry. Available at: http://www.nature.com/ebd/about.html. Accessed 04/23/08.
3. J Evid Based Dent Pract. Available at: http://journals.elsevierhealth.com/periodicals/ymed/home. Accessed 05/29/08.
4. Guyatt G, Rennie D. Users' guides to the medical literature. JAMA 1993;270(17):2096–7.
5. Oxman A, Sackett D, Guyatt G. Users' guides to the medical literature. I. How to get started. The Evidence-Based Medicine Working Group. JAMA 1993;270(17):2093–5.
6. Guyatt G, Haynes R, Jaeschke R, et al. Users' guides to the medical literature. XXV. Evidence-Based medicine: principles for applying the users' guides to patient care. Evidence-Based Medicine Working Group. JAMA 2000;284(10):1290–6.
7. Sackett D, Straus S. Finding and applying evidence during clinical rounds: the "evidence cart". JAMA 1998;280(15):1336–8.
8. Richards D, Lawrence A. Evidence based dentistry. Braz Dent J 1995;179:270–3.
9. McCulloch C. Can evidence-based dental health care assure quality? J Dent Educ 1994;58:654–6.
10. Reekie D. The future of dentistry—the evidence revolution. Braz Dent J 1998;184:262–3.
11. Haynes R, Davis D, McKibbon A, et al. A critical appraisal of the efficacy of continuing medical education. JAMA 1984;251:61–4.
12. Bader J. A review of evaluations of effectiveness in continuing dental education. Möbius 1987;7:39–48.
13. Bedos C, Allison P. Are the results of dental research accessible to Canadian dentists? J Can Dent Assoc 2002;68:602–5.
14. Richards D. Integrating evidence-based teaching into to clinical practice should improve outcomes. Evid Based Dent 2005;6:47.
15. Iqbal A, Glenny AM. General dental practitioners' knowledge of and attitudes towards evidence based practice. Braz Dent J 2002;193(10):587–91.
16. Watt R, McGlone P, Evans D, et al. The facilitating factors and barriers influencing change in dental practice in a sample of English general dental practitioners. Braz Dent J 2004;197(8):485–9.
17. Schleyer TK, Thyvalikakath TP, Spallek H, et al. Clinical computing in general dentistry. J Am Med Inform Assoc 2006;13(3):344–52.
18. Cochrane Oral Health Group. Reviews. Available at: http://www.ohg.cochrane.org/reviews.html. Accessed 04/11/08.

19. Beirne P, Worthington HV, Clarkson JE. Routine scale and polish for periodontal health in adults. [Reviews]. Cochrane Database of Systematic Reviews 2007;4: CD004625. DOI: 10.1002/14651858.CD004625.pub3.

20. Beirne P, Clarkson JE, Worthington HV. Recall intervals for oral health in primary care patients. Reviews. Cochrane Database of Systematic Reviews 2007;4: CD004346. DOI: 10.1002/14651858.CD004346.pub3.

21. Montenegro R, Needleman I, Moles D, et al. Quality of RCTs in periodontology—a systematic review. J Dent Res 2002;81(12):866–70.

22. Iqbal MK, Kim S. For teeth requiring endodontic treatment, what are the differences in outcomes of restored endodontically treated teeth compared to implant-supported restorations? Int J Oral Maxillofac Implants 2007;22(Suppl): 96–116.

23. Torabinejad M, Anderson P, Bader J, et al. Outcomes of root canal treatment and restoration, implant-supported single crowns, fixed partial dentures, and extraction without replacement: a systematic review. J Prosthet Dent 2007;98(4): 285–311.

24. Beauchamp J, Caufield PW, Crall JJ, et al. Evidence-based clinical recommendations for the use of pit-and-fissure sealants: a report of the American Dental Association council on scientific affairs. J Am Dent Assoc 2008;139(3):257–68.

25. Griffin SO, Oong E, Kohn W, et al. The effectiveness of sealants in managing caries lesions. J Dent Res 2008;87(2):169–74.

26. Dental Practice-Based Research Network. Available at: http://www.dentalpbrn. org/home.asp. Accessed 05/29/08.

27. Pearl Network. Available at: https://web.emmes.com/study/pearl/index.htm. Accessed 05/29/08.

28. Precedent. Available at: https://workbench.axioresearch.com/NWPrecedent/index.htm. Accessed 05/29/08.

29. Fontana M, Zero D. Bridging the gap in caries management between research and practice through education: the Indiana University experience. J Dent Educ 2007;71:579–91.

30. Azarpazhooh A, Mayhall JT, Leake JL. Introducing dental students to evidence-based decisions in dental care. J Dent Educ 2008;72:87–109.

31. Bahrami M, Deery C, Clarkson JE, et al. Effectiveness of strategies to disseminate and implement clinical guidelines for the management of impacted and unerupted third molars in primary dental care, a cluster randomised controlled trial. Braz Dent J 2004;197(11):691–6.

32. van der Sanden WJ, Mettes DG, Plasschaert AJ, et al. Effectiveness of clinical practice guideline implementation on lower third molar management in improving clinical decision-making: a randomized controlled trial. Eur J Oral Sci 2005; 113(5):349–54.

33. O'Brien K, Wright J, Conboy F, et al. The effect of orthodontic referral guidelines: a randomised controlled trial. Braz Dent J 2000;188(7):392–7.

34. Yogi Berra. Wikiquote. Available at: http://en.wikiquote.org/wiki/Yogi_Berra. Accessed 05/29/08.

35. Website on Evidence-Based Dentistry, American Dental Association. Available at: http://ada.org/prof/resources/ebd/index.asp.

36. Gavrvin J. EBD Champions. ADA News 2008;39(10):8–9,12.

37. Rindal DB, Rush WA, Boyle RG. Clinical inertia in dentistry: a review of the phenomenon. J Contemp Dent Pract 2008;9(1):113–21.

Evidence-Based Dentistry and the Concept of Harm

Mark V. Thomas, DMD[a],*, Sharon E. Straus, MD[b]

- Evidence-based dentistry • Evidence-based practice
- Evidence-based medicine • Risk • Informed consent
- Risk management • Alendronate • Osteonecrosis

Evidence-based medicine (EBM) is "the conscientious, explicit, and judicious use of current best evidence in making decisions about the care of individual patients."[1] It requires the integration of best research evidence with the clinician's expertise and the patient's unique values and circumstances. One of the most important issues in deciding what course of treatment to select is balancing the potential risks and benefits of treatment. A framework for evidence-based decision-making includes formulating the clinical question and then retrieving, appraising, and considering the applicability of the evidence to the patient.

CLINICAL SCENARIO

To illustrate the process of using evidence-based medicine to quantify harm, consider the following clinical scenario. A 62-year-old postmenopausal woman has recently been diagnosed with generalized chronic periodontitis of advanced severity. She has recently received nonsurgical therapy (ie, scaling and root planing, oral hygiene, re-evaluation of treatment response), but problems persist at some sites (eg, bleeding, attachment loss, and probing depths ≥6 mm) and the general dentist has referred the patient to you, the periodontist, for evaluation and treatment. The dentist has suggested that surgical debridement may be indicated in the posterior sextants of the patient's mouth. You examine the patient and concur with the dentist's assessment. However, there is a complicating factor in this patient's history. She has osteoporosis, for which she has taken alendronate for 5 years. Bisphosphonates (BPs), including alendronate, have been associated with osteonecrosis of the jaws, a condition often referred to as "bisphosphonate-related osteonecrosis of the jaws" (BRONJ).[2–4] While

---

[a] Department of Oral Health Practice, Division of Periodontology, University of Kentucky College of Dentistry, 800 Rose Street, Room M-122, Lexington, KY 40536-0297, USA
[b] Faculty of Medicine, University of Toronto, Toronto, Ontario M5S 1A8, Canada
* Corresponding author.
E-mail address: mvthom0@email.uky.edu (M. V. Thomas).

Dent Clin N Am 53 (2009) 23–32
doi:10.1016/j.cden.2008.11.002   dental.theclinics.com
0011-8532/08/$ – see front matter © 2009 Elsevier Inc. All rights reserved.

this has been a rare occurrence, the consequences have been catastrophic in some cases. A recent study reported that repeated surgical interventions were required in more than 25% of patients suffering from BRONJ.[5] Some patients have required aggressive (and occasionally disfiguring) surgeries, such as partial maxillectomy and mandibulectomy, sometimes with serious sequelae, such as septic shock.[4,6,7] Given this situation, what information do you need to adequately advise your patient about the risks and benefits of treatment for her condition?

This evidence-based decision-making process includes consideration of (1) the risks associated with the procedure (viz, open flap debridement), (2) the risks associated with alternative treatment (eg, additional nonsurgical therapy with or without adjunctive aids, such as antibiotics), and (3) the risk of periodontal infection in the absence of treatment. With regard to the potential risk of BRONJ posed by nonsurgical therapy or untreated periodontal disease, there is insufficient evidence to assess this risk. There are no reports of BRONJ subsequent to nonsurgical periodontal therapy, and while there are reports of BRONJ occurring in the absence of dental treatment, there is little data on the presence of pre-existing periodontal disease as a risk factor. One group has reported periodontal disease as a comorbidity in 84% of a series of 119 cases of BRONJ.[4] However, the investigators do not define what constitutes periodontitis. They do report severe periodontitis as a precipitating factor in 28% of their cases, but it is not clear whether the periodontitis was in conjunction with other risk factors or not. It is of interest that approximately 25% of their cases occurred in the absence of precipitating dental intervention or trauma. The cases reported are a composite of patients referred to the investigators surgical service and "43 cases well documented by colleagues." This study constitutes a rather low level of evidence. Thus, the inivestigators can make no inferences as to whether untreated periodontal disease might predispose to BRONJ. The risk of no intervention is probably not zero, but it is unknown.

In order to provide optimal care for our hypothetical patient, we must find evidence that will allow us to quantify the risk of BRONJ subsequent to periodontal surgery. We will do this by locating and evaluating high-quality evidence relating to this question. Following an appraisal of the evidence, we will be better prepared to advise our patient, who can decide what option is best for her.

FINDING THE EVIDENCE

Based on the scenario, we have posed the following question: what is the risk of BRONJ in a postmenopausal woman who has taken alendronate for 5 years. To answer the question, we must match the question to the appropriate study type. Since this is a question of harm, it is best addressed by a systematic review of randomized trials or a single large randomized trial. As reported elsewhere in this issue (Thomas and colleagues), evidence can be ranked on the basis of quality. For therapy questions, systematic reviews and meta-analyses combine results from a number of randomized, controlled trials (RCTs) and, therefore, are regarded as the highest quality evidence, assuming the studies were well-designed and had adequate statistical power to detect differences between modalities. It is common to speak of a "hierarchy" of evidence,[8] often depicted in the form of a pyramid such as the "5S" model proposed by Haynes (**Fig. 1**).[9]

Note in **Fig. 1** that individual studies are to be found at the lowest level of the pyramid. Obviously, individual RCTs are the bedrock or foundation of the pyramid, but evidence is strengthened when it is based upon syntheses of a number of well-designed studies. Systematic reviews are syntheses based on the results of multiple

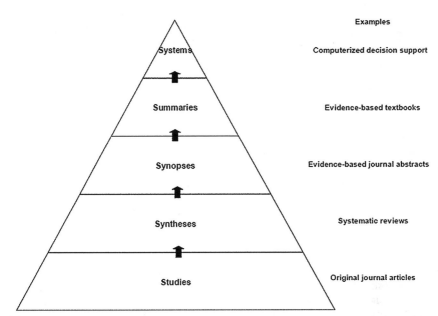

Fig. 1. Five levels of evidence. (*From* Haynes GB. Of studies, syntheses, synopses, summaries, and systems: the "5S" evolution of information services for evidence-based health care decisions. ACP Journal Club 2006;145(3):A–8; with permission.)

RCTs. Such reviews may be found in various repositories, the most well known of which is the Cochrane Library (www.cochane.org). Other sources of evidence are listed in **Figs. 2** and **3**. A systematic review is a comprehensive search of the literature on a specific question. In this process, there are explicit inclusion and exclusion criteria used to determine what studies should be included in the analysis, as well as an explicit description of the search methodology and results.[10] The meta-analysis is a statistical synthesis of the data from several studies of similar design, with studies weighted with regard to sample size. It is often of value when several RCTs have been performed which, individually, lack the statistical power to detect statistically significant differences between interventions, but are capable of doing so in the aggregate.[11]

"Synopses" refer to brief critical analyses of original articles and reviews that are found in evidence-based journals, such as *The Journal of Evidence-Based Dental Practice* or the *ACP Journal Club*. The next level includes summaries, which integrate the best evidence from the lower levels (relying on systematic reviews whenever possible). Summaries integrate the whole spectrum of evidence concerning the management of a particular health issue, such as colon cancer, periodontitis, or metabolic syndrome. Such a summary brings together evidence from individual studies, systematic reviews, and synopses in one compiled and easily accessible source. Of course, it is necessary that the user of such evidence must exercise due diligence by critically appraising the methodology used to create the summary. This appraisal "should include details of the retrieval process used to find best evidence, the appraisal process for rating the quality of evidence should be explicit and auditable, [and] key references provided for all care recommendations."[9]

There is one level beyond the summary. Clinical-decision support systems link the patient's electronic health record to current best-evidence based on the individual

Summaries of Systematic Reviews

Resource	Link	Information Available
EBD at ADA.org	www.ada.org/goto/ebd	Summaries of dental systematic reviews published elsewhere (new ADA-sponsored critical summaries are under development); additional Web resources
Journal of Evidence-Based Dental Practice	http://journals.elsevierhealth.com/periodicals/ymed	Summaries of dental systematic reviews, plus commentary and analysis; critical evaluations of published articles on various topics
Database of Abstracts of Reviews of Effectiveness (DARE)	http://www.crd.york.ac.uk/CRDWeb/	Structured abstracts of systematic reviews; includes commentary on overall review quality
National Library for Health—Oral Health Specialist Library	http://www.library.nhs.uk/oralhealth/	Structured abstracts of systematic reviews
Evidence-Based Dentistry journal (UK)	http://www.nature.com/ebd/archive/index.html	Systematic review summaries/analyses.
Evidentista (Pan American Centers for Evidence-Based Dentistry)	http://us.evidentista.org/?o=1026	Clinical questions and answers grouped by topic area
Agency for Healthcare Research and Quality (AHRQ)	http://www.ahrq.gov/clinic/epcquick.htm	Summaries of AHRQ evidence reports on dental caries, dental patients who are HIV positive, scaling and root planning therapy, and others
Bandolier: Dental and Oral Health	http://www.jr2.ox.ac.uk/bandolier/booth/booths/dental.html	Critical appraisals of systematic reviews and supporting studies on dental topics
Cochrane Oral Health Group	http://www.ohg.cochrane.org/reviews.html	Abstracts and plain-language summaries of dental systematic reviews
Centre for Evidence-Based Dentistry	http://www.cebd.org/?o=1069	Evidence summaries from the Oral Health Specialist library grouped by topic and/or specialty area

Clinical Recommendations/Guidelines

Resource	Link	Information Available
National Guideline Clearinghouse	www.guidelines.gov	Clinical practice guidelines
ADA Evidence-Based Clinical Recommendations	http://www.ada.org/prof/resources/ebd/clinical.asp	Evidence-based clinical recommendations on oral health topics, including topical fluoride and sealants
PubMed Clinical Queries (National Library of Medicine)	http://www.ncbi.nlm.nih.gov/entrez/query/static/clinical.shtml#reviews	Clinical practice guidelines grouped by category
National Institute for Health and Clinical Excellence (NICE)	http://www.nice.org.uk/guidance/index.jsp?action=byTopic&o=7298&set=true	Clinical guidelines from UK on dental recall
Centers for Disease Control and Prevention (CDC) Division of Oral Health	http://www.cdc.gov/oralhealth/guidelines.htm	Guidelines developed by CDC and the Task Force on Community Preventive Services
Scottish Intercollegiate Guidelines Network	http://www.sign.ac.uk/guidelines/published/index.html#Dentistry	Clinical guidelines on dental topics available as full guidelines and in quick reference guide format
Royal College of Surgeons (RCS) of England	http://www.rcseng.ac.uk/fds/clinical_guidelines	Clinical guidelines on common clinical situations
Agency for Healthcare Research and Quality (AHRQ)	http://www.ahrq.gov/clinic/cpgsix.htm	Clinical practice guidelines from the National Guideline Clearinghouse, Department of Health and Human Services, and AHRQ
SUMSearch	http://sumsearch.uthscsa.edu/	Searches free online resources—PubMed (Medline), Database of Abstracts of Reviews of Effectiveness (DARE), National Institutes of Health (NIH) Guidelines Clearinghouse—to retrieve systematic reviews and/or clinical guidelines.
Centre for Evidence-Based Dentistry	http://www.cebd.org/?o=1069	Guidelines and consensus statements

Systematic Reviews

Resource	Link	Information Available
EBD at ADA.org	www.ada.org/goto/ebd	Abstracts of published systematic reviews on dental topics grouped by clinical topic areas, listed in A-Z format; full text available for systematic reviews published by the *Journal of the American Dental Association*
Cochrane Oral Health Group (affiliated with the Cochrane Collaboration)	http://www.ohg.cochrane.org/reviews.html#reviews	Systematic reviews from the Cochrane Oral Health Group
PubMed systematic review search page	http://www.ncbi.nlm.nih.gov/entrez/query/static/clinical.shtml#reviews	Systematic review abstracts, plus links to full-text copies where available.
EviDents Search Engine for EBD	http://medinformatics.uthscsa.edu/EviDents/	Searchable resource for systematic review abstracts and other studies
TRIP Database, Oral Health page	http://www.tripdatabase.com/oral/specialismhomepage.html	Systematic reviews related to oral health
SUMSearch	http://sumsearch.uthscsa.edu/	Searches free online resources—PubMed (Medline), Database of Abstracts of Reviews of Effectiveness (DARE), NIH Guidelines Clearinghouse—to retrieve systematic reviews and/or clinical guidelines
International Centre for Evidence-Based Oral Health (Eastman Dental Institute, UK)	http://www.eastman.ucl.ac.uk/~pdarkins/iceph/	"Publications" link includes full-text systematic reviews on clinical topics
Google Scholar	http://scholar.google.com/	Search tool for systematic reviews and other research
Centre for Evidence-Based Dentistry	http://www.cebd.org/?o=1069	Resources on dental systematic reviews
AHRQ Evidence-based Practice Center (EPC) Reports	http://www.ahrq.gov/clinic/epcindex.htm#oral	Evidence-based reports on oral health topics
Netting the Evidence	http://www.google.com/coop/cse?cx=004326897958477606950%3Adjcbsrxkatm	Customized Google search engine devoted to evidence-based practice

Fig. 2. Sources of evidence. (*Courtesy of* the American Dental Association. Copyright © ADA; used with permission.)

Evidence-Based Centers

Centre for Evidence-Based Dentistry	http://www.cebd.org/
Centre for Evidence-Based Medicine (Oxford University)	www.cebm.net
Cochrane Collaboration	http://www.thecochranelibrary.com
Agency for Healthcare Research and Quality	http://www.ahrq.gov/clinic/epcix.htm
DSM-Forsyth Center for Evidence-Based Dentistry	http://www.forsyth.org/forsyth.asp?pg=100111
Centre for Health Evidence	http://www.cche.net/
International Centre for Evidence-Based Oral Health (Eastman Dental Institute—London, UK)	http://www.eastman.ucl.ac.uk/~pdarkins/iceph/
Evidentista (Pan American Centers for Evidence-Based Dentistry)	http://us.evidentista.org/?o=1026
Centre for Evidence-Based Medicine (University of Toronto, Canada)	http://www.cebm.utoronto.ca/

Journals

Journal of Evidence-Based Dental Practice	http://www.elsevier.com/wps/find/journaldescription.cws_home/623234/description#description
Evidence-Based Dentistry	http://www.nature.com/ebd/index.html
Evidence-Based Medicine Online	http://ebm.bmjjournals.com/

Databases

Cochrane Library	http://www.thecochranelibrary.com
PubMed (National Library of Medicine)	http://www.pubmed.com
TRIP Database, Oral Health page	http://www.tripdatabase.com/oral/specialismhomepage.html
Database of Abstracts of Reviews of Effectiveness (DARE)	http://www.crd.york.ac.uk/crdweb/
National Guideline Clearinghouse	www.guidelines.gov

Other Resources

Evidence-Based Dentistry Resource Guide (Virginia Commonwealth University)	http://www.library.vcu.edu/tml/bibs/ebd.html
Evidence-Based Medicine Resource Center	http://www.ebmny.org/
Evidence-Based On Call	http://www.eboncall.org/
Health Evidence Bulletins-Wales (oral health)	http://hebw.cf.ac.uk/oralhealth/index.html
PrimeAnswers	http://www.primeanswers.org/primeanswers/index.cfm

Tutorials

ScHARR Introduction to Evidence-based Practice on the Internet	http://www.shef.ac.uk/scharr/ir/netting/
Evidence-Based Clinical Practice Tutorial (Miner Library)	http://www.urmc.rochester.edu/hslt/miner/resources/evidence_based/index.cfm
A Student's Guide to the Medical Literature (University of Colorado Health Sciences Center)	http://grinch.uchsc.edu/sg/index.html
Evidence-Based Medicine: Finding the Best Clinical Literature (University of Illinois Library of the Health Sciences)	http://www.uic.edu/depts/lib/lhsp/resources/ebm.shtml
Introduction to Evidence-Based Medicine (Duke University Medical Center Library and Health Sciences Library, UNC-Chapel Hill)	http://www.hsl.unc.edu/services/tutorials/ebm/index.htm
PubMed Tutorial	http://www.nlm.nih.gov/bsd/disted/pubmed.html
Using Numerical Results from Systematic Reviews in Clinical Practice	http://www.annals.org/cgi/content/full/126/9/712
SUNY Downstate Medical Center Evidence-Based Medicine Tutorial	http://library.downstate.edu/EBM2/contents.htm

(Continued)

Fig. 3. Other EBD/EBM resources. (*Courtesy of* the American Dental Association. Copyright © ADA; used with permission.)

patient's clinical circumstances. There are few such systems currently available, and those that exist are limited in their scope and have proven imperfect in application.[12] However, the pieces are in place that can make the continued evolution of such systems likely.

In the case study described above, we could locate no summaries or synopses that addressed our question, so an initial search was conducted in the Cochrane Library, using the search terms "bisphosphonate" AND "oral" OR "jaw." Three recent reviews were found. Wells and colleagues[13] analyzed results of seven trials involving 14,000 women in which risedronate was compared with a placebo. The investigators report that "[f]or adverse events, no statistically significant differences were found in any of the included studies. *However, observational data has led to concerns regarding the*

Resources for Critical Appraisal and Evidence Analysis

Appraisal Tools—Critical Appraisal Skills Programme (CASP)	http://www.phru.nhs.uk/Pages/PHD/resources.htm
AMSTAR (tool for the "assessment of multiple systematic reviews")	http://www.biomedcentral.com/1471-2288/7/10
Grading of Recommendations, Assessment, Development and Evaluation (GRADE) Working Group publications	http://www.gradeworkinggroup.org/index.htm
QUOROM Statement ("Quality of Reporting of Meta-Analyses")	http://www.consort-statement.org/index.aspx?o=1346
Center for Evidence-Based Medicine, Critical Appraisal Tools	http://www.cebm.net/index.aspx?o=1023
CONSORT Statement (consolidated standards of reporting trials)	http://www.consort-statement.org/
Meta-analysis of Observational Studies in Epidemiology (MOOSE): A Proposal for Reporting	http://jama.ama-assn.org/cgi/content/full/283/15/2008

Glossaries of Terms

American Dental Association EBD Glossary of Terms	http://www.ada.org/prof/resources/ebd/glossary.asp
Bandolier EBM Glossary	http://www.jr2.ox.ac.uk/bandolier/glossary.html
British Medical Journal—Clinical Evidence Glossary	http://clinicalevidence.bmj.com/ceweb/resources/glossary.jsp
Centre for Evidence-Based Medicine: Key Terms in Evidence-Based Practice	http://www.cebm.net/index.aspx?o=1116
Evidence-Based On Call (Glossary)	http://www.eboncall.org/CONTENT/glossary.htm
Definitions of Evidence-Based Practice (University of Sheffield, UK)	http://www.shef.ac.uk/scharr/ir/def.html

Fig. 3. (continued)

potential risk for upper gastrointestinal injury and, less commonly, osteonecrosis of the jaw" (emphasis added). Note that the investigators are not referring to their reviewed trials when discussing the possibility of osteonecrosis but to other published cases and case series. This review represents a very high level of evidence. Another review (by the same investigators) examined 11 trials of alendronate involving over 12,000 women.[14,15] Again, there was no statistical difference between the adverse events seen in the test and placebo arms, although the investigators also report the caveat noted above regarding observational studies. This study is even more relevant to the patient in the case study, because subjects in the test arm were administered the same bisphosphonate that the patient in the case study is taking.

The third review in the Cochrane examined 21 RCTs of intravenous bisphosphonate use in metastatic breast cancer.[16] Again, no serious adverse effects were noted, but the investigators include the caveat that BRONJ has been reported in subsequent case reports and observational studies. Thus, no cases of BRONJ were reported in the trials reviewed in these systematic reviews. These reviews represent a high level of evidence and are based upon collectively large sample sizes. Two of the studies, representing results of over 26,000 osteoporotic subjects, reported no adverse events related to osteonecrosis; however, others have suggested the possibility of under-reporting of BRONJ.[17] Walter and colleagues[17] report a much higher incidence of BRONJ in their population, but it should be noted that these were patients with metastatic prostatic carcinoma receiving intravenous BPs (as opposeed to oral bisphosphonates, such as our patient is taking).

The systematic reviews discussed above represent a very high level of evidence. However, there is some evidence (although of a much lower level of quality and/or applicability to our patient) that suggests there is a risk of BRONJ subsequent to dental surgery. While this evidence is not as compelling, it is presented for the sake of completeness. Using PubMed, another search was undertaken using the search terms "bisphosphonate" and "jaw." The initial search was limited to RCTs. Four citations were returned, two of which were somewhat relevant to the question. The first was a prospective trial of 7714 osteoporotic women treated with intravenous zole-dronic acid.[18] In that study, only two cases of osteonecrosis were noted, one of which occurred in a patient taking the placebo. Both cases resolved with antibiotics or debridement. This trial is significant because the study population consisted of post-menopausal osteoporotic women, rather than patients with metastic cancer. It is likely that this population is more closely related to the case-study patient's situation. A second trial involved the use of zoledronic acid in cases of asymptomatic myeloma, which is clearly less relevant to the case-study patient.[19] Musto and colleagues[19] reported on results of a trial of 163 patients, of whom 81 received zoledronic acid. One case of osteonecrosis was observed, for an incidence of 1.2%. Again, however, these myeloma patients may differ in important ways from case-study patient and the results may not be applicable to osteoporotic patients.

One report raised the possibility of under-reporting of BRONJ in RCTs. Walter and colleagues[17] carefully examined a group of 43 patients being treated with BPs for metastatic prostatic carcinoma. They reported that 18% of these patients developed BRONJ and suggest the possibility that the incidence of the condition might be under-reported. This prospective study was unique in that the subjects received careful oral examinations for evidence of dental pathology and, specifically, osteonecrotic lesions. It has been reported that adverse events are often under-reported in clinical trials. Papanikolaou and Ioannidis[20] reviewed 1,727 systematic reviews and found that only 138 included evidence on greater than or equal to 4,000 subjects. This is the minimum sample size required for adequate power to detect an intervention-related adverse effect in 1% of subjects.

Another PubMed search was undertaken, using the search terms "bisphospho-nate" and "jaw," but without any limits. A total of 304 citations were retrieved, most of which were related to the treatment of metastatic bone cancer and were not felt to be entirely relevant to the case-study patient's situation. One large systematic review was identified that assessed the effectiveness of alendronate in fracture prevention in osteoporotic women.[21] These investigators reviewed 11 trials represent-ing approximately 12,000 women. They stated that "[f]or adverse events, the authors found no statistically significant difference in any included study." They did include the caveat that "observational data raise concerns about potential risk for upper gastro-intestinal injury and, less commonly, osteonecrosis of the jaw."

Finally, a PubMed search was conducted using the search terms "periodontal surgery" and "bisphosphonate." Four citations were returned. One was a general narrative review in Japanese and was not deemed relevant. One described the use of a bisphosphonate in preventing bone loss in an animal model. A third was a case report of a patient who experienced a nonhealing osteonecrotic lesion following peri-odontal surgery in a 78-year-old woman who had taken an oral bisphosphonate for 5 years. The last was a series of 119 cases reported by Marx and colleagues[3] and cited previously. Marx and colleagues reported the following "inciting events" in their case series: 25% were spontaneous and no precipitating event could be identified, 38% were because of removal of teeth, 29% were because of advanced periodontitis (case definition not provided), and 11% were because of periodontal surgery. As noted above, this study represents a low level of evidence, but does suggest that there may be some risk of BRONJ associated with both periodontal infection and peri-odontal surgery.

Collectively, this "secondary" evidence is much less impressive than the results of the large systematic reviews found in the Cochrane Library. However, given the poten-tial serious nature of BRONJ, it seems reasonable to acknowledge the existence of this additional evidence.

EVALUATING THE EVIDENCE

At this point, it may be concluded that there may be a small, but finite risk of a potentially serious complication subsequent to periodontal surgery in patients taking alendronate. There may also be a small risk of osteonecrotic lesions in patients suffering from advanced periodontitis, but there is insufficient evidence to quantify this risk.

Ideally, we would like to communicate this risk to our patient in a way that is easily understood. This is most easily done by calculating a "number needed to harm" (NNH), which is specific for this treatment in this type of patient. Specifically, the NNH is that number of patients who would need to be treated before one case of BRONJ was seen.[22] If the evidence is limited to only the highest quality (the systematic reviews in the Cochrane Library),[13,15] one would conclude that the NNH is infinity, for no cases of BRONJ were reported in any of the trials that were reviewed. Nevertheless, there are some case reports and some of these cases have had serious sequelae. As noted earlier, it is possible that BRONJ cases were not captured because of insufficient length of follow-up or failure to see this as an adverse event related to the BP therapy.

On the other hand, there is no evidence implicating nonsurgical therapy in BRONJ. Given the possibility of arresting her disease with further nonsurgical treatment, and the absence of evidence that nonsurgical therapy is a risk factor for BRONJ, and the slowly progressive nature of periodontitis, it may make sense to recommend further nonsurgical treatment for the patient. For example, some additional scaling and root planing might be performed, locally delivered controlled-release antibiotics could be used, and more frequent maintenance debridement might occur. Periodontal disease is often slowly progressive and the patient's condition can be easily assessed at each maintenance visit. Of course, it is necessary to tell the patient that there is some evidence (albeit weak) that suggests that periodontal infections may contribute to the pathogenesis of BRONJ and the magnitude of that risk is also unknown.

Hippocrates suggested that the goal of medicine was to "first, do no harm." Unfortunately, there are no interventions that are free of risk. Implicit in most treatments is the possibility of harm. This can range from the trivial, such as mild discomfort following venipuncture, to the life-changing (such as iatrogenic nerve damage to the facial nerve following parotid surgery), to life-ending. Although it is not possible to provide most treatments without some risk, it is the clinician's duty to reduce such risk and to provide honest estimates of the negative consequences of treatment (eg, NNT), so that patients can make rational decisions regarding their care. We must be as zealous in describing our failures as we are our successes, so that we can learn to avoid them or, at least, minimize their consequences. Evidence-based health care provides the tools to move toward this goal.

SUMMARY

It is sobering, but important, that clinicians reflect on the fact that some patients are left in a worse condition after treatment than they were before treatment. It is the duty of all health care providers to reduce patient risk by selecting appropriate therapies and informing patients of unavoidable risks. In this way, we can fulfill our duty to our patients. EBM provides a basis by which we can evaluate the risks of various therapeutic options and communicate this information to our patients in a way that is useful and easily understood.

REFERENCES

1. Sackett DL, Rosenberg WM, Gray JA, et al. Evidence based medicine: what it is and what it isn't. BMJ 1996;312(7023):71–2.

2. Woo SB, Hellstein JW, Kalmar JR. Narrative [corrected] review: bisphosphonates and osteonecrosis of the jaws. Ann Intern Med 2006;144(10):753–61.
3. Marx RE, Cillo JE Jr, Ulloa JJ. Oral bisphosphonate-induced osteonecrosis: risk factors, prediction of risk using serum CTX testing, prevention, and treatment. J Oral Maxillofac Surg 2007;65(12):2397–410.
4. Marx RE, Sawatari Y, Fortin M, et al. Bisphosphonate-induced exposed bone (osteonecrosis/osteopetrosis) of the jaws: risk factors, recognition, prevention, and treatment. J Oral Maxillofac Surg 2005;63(11):1567–75.
5. Eckert AW, Maurer P, Meyer L, et al. Bisphosphonate-related jaw necrosis— severe complication in maxillofacial surgery. Cancer Treat Rev 2007;33(1): 58–63.
6. La Verde N, Bareggi C, Garassino M, et al. Osteonecrosis of the jaw (ONJ) in cancer patients treated with bisphosphonates: how the knowledge of a phenomenon can change its evolution. Support Care Cancer 2008;16(11):1311–5.
7. Ripamonti CI, Maniezzo M, Campa T, et al. Decreased occurrence of osteonecrosis of the jaw after implementation of dental preventive measures in solid tumour patients with bone metastases treated with bisphosphonates. The experience of the National Cancer Institute of Milan. Annals of Oncology. E-pub July 22, 2008. doi:10.1093/annonc/mdn526.
8. McKibbon A, Wyer P, Jaeschke R, et al. Finding the evidence. In: Guyatt G, Rennie D, Meade MO, et al, editors. Users' Guides to the Medical Literature. New York: McGraw-Hill Medical; 2008. p. 29–58.
9. Haynes RB. Of studies, syntheses, synopses, summaries, and systems: the "5S" evolution of information services for evidence-based health care decisions. ACP J Club 2006;145(3):A8–9.
10. Guyatt G, Jaeschke R, Prasad K, et al. Summarizing the evidence. In: Guyatt G, Rennie D, Meade MO, et al, editors. Users' Guides to the Medical Literature. New York: McGraw-Hill Medical; 2008. p. 523–54.
11. Last JM. A Dictionary of Epidemiology. Oxford: Oxford University Press; 2001.
12. Garg AX, Adhikari NK, McDonald H, et al. Effects of computerized clinical decision support systems on practitioner performance and patient outcomes: a systematic review. JAMA 2005;293(10):1223–38.
13. Hujoel PP. Definitive vs. exploratory periodontal trials: a survey of published studies. J Dent Res 1995;74(8):1453–8.
14. Hujoel PP, DeRouen TA. A survey of endpoint characteristics in periodontal clinical trials published 1988–1992, and implications for future studies. J Clin Periodontol 1995;22(5):397–407.
15. Wells G, Cranney A, Peterson J, et al. Risedronate for the primary and secondary prevention of osteoporotic fractures in postmenopausal women. Cochrane Database Syst Rev 2008;(1):CD004523.
16. Cranney A, Wells G, Willan A, et al. Meta-analyses of therapies for postmenopausal osteoporosis. II. Meta-analysis of alendronate for the treatment of postmenopausal women. Endocr Rev 2002;23(4):508–16.
17. Wells GA, Cranney A, Peterson J, et al. Alendronate for the primary and secondary prevention of osteoporotic fractures in postmenopausal women. Cochrane Database Syst Rev 2008;(1):CD001155.
18. Pavlakis N, Schmidt R, Stockler M. Bisphosphonates for breast cancer. Cochrane Database Syst Rev 2005;(3):CD003474.
19. Walter C, Al-Nawas B, Grotz KA, et al. Prevalence and risk factors of bisphosphonate-associated osteonecrosis of the jaw in prostate cancer patients with advanced disease treated with zoledronate. Eur Urol 2008;54(5):1066–72.

20. Grbic JT, Landesberg R, Lin SQ, et al. Incidence of osteonecrosis of the jaw in women with postmenopausal osteoporosis in the health outcomes and reduced incidence with zoledronic acid once yearly pivotal fracture trial. J Am Dent Assoc 2008;139(1):32–40.

21. Musto P, Petrucci MT, Bringhen S, et al. A multicenter, randomized clinical trial comparing zoledronic acid versus observation in patients with asymptomatic myeloma. Cancer 2008;113(7):1588–95.

22. Papanikolaou PN, Ioannidis JP. Availability of large-scale evidence on specific harms from systematic reviews of randomized trials. Am J Med 2004;117(8): 582–9.

The Benefits of Evidence-Based Dentistry for the Private Dental Office

Jane Gillette, DDS[a], Joseph D. Matthews, DDS, MSc[b],
Julie Frantsve-Hawley, PhD[c], Robert J. Weyant, DMD, DrPH[d,*]

KEYWORDS

- Evidence-based medicine • Practice management
- Dental • Dental offices

Dentistry, like other health care fields, is a science-based profession. As such, it is expected that research and technologies will continually evolve based on advances in the understanding of the science, and that the corresponding treatment decisions will evolve as well. Practitioners are continually challenged with the task of keeping current with the scientific literature. Given the sheer volume of scientific journal articles and the wide variations in methodology, meeting this challenge continues to be difficult for all health care professionals.

During the 1990s, a new process for incorporating the most current scientific literature into health care emerged. Known as evidence-based medicine (EBM), this process was developed as a systematic approach to identify and critically assess the evidence relevant to specific clinical questions. The ultimate purpose of EBM is to help health care providers implement the most current scientific information into patient care.

The term *evidence-based medicine* first appeared in the medical literature in 1992.[1] In 1995, Dr. David Sackett founded the Oxford Centre for Evidence-Based Medicine[2] and is often credited with early advances in the EBM movement. In a 1996 *British Medical Journal* article, Sackett provided the most commonly cited and used definition of evidence-based medicine (**Box 1**).[3] Sackett acknowledged that EBM requires

[a] Northwest Practice-based REsearch Collaborative in Evidence-based DENTistry, 2055 North 22nd Avenue, Ste 3, Bozeman, MT 59718, USA
[b] University of New Mexico, School of Medicine, 3500 Trinity Drive, Suite B-2, Los Alamos, New Mexico 87544, USA
[c] Research Institute and Center for Evidence-based Dentistry, American Dental Association, 211 East, Chicago Avenue, Chicago, IL 60611, USA
[d] Department of Dental Public Health and Information Management, School of Dental Medicine, University of Pittsburgh, Pittsburgh, PA 15261, USA
* Corresponding author.
E-mail address: rjw1@pitt.edu (R. J. Weyant).

Dent Clin N Am 53 (2009) 33–45
doi:10.1016/j.cden.2008.09.002
0011-8532/08/$ – see front matter © 2009 Elsevier Inc. All rights reserved.

> **Box 1**
> **Sackett definition of EBM**
>
> Evidence-based medicine is the conscientious, explicit, and judicious use of current best evidence in making decisions about the care of individual patients. The practice of evidence-based medicine means integrating individual clinical expertise with the best available external clinical evidence from systematic research.
>
> *Data from* Sackett DL, Rosenberg WM, Gray JA, et al. Evidence based medicine: What it is and what it isn't. BMJ 1996;312(7023):71–2.

the incorporation of three key items into the clinical decision-making process: the best evidence, clinical expertise, and patient values.[4]

These same three elements form the foundation for evidence-based approaches to health care by many professional groups, including dentistry. In the fall of 2001, the American Dental Association (ADA) adopted an evidence-based dentistry policy statement, which includes the same three elements—scientific evidence, clinical expertise, and the patient's needs and preferences—in the definition of evidence-based dentistry (EBD) (**Box 2**). By systematically incorporating the best available clinical evidence, the evidence-based approach aims to help dental professionals apply their professional judgment to make the best-informed clinical decisions. The policy statement also emphasizes that scientific evidence, by itself, cannot dictate patient care, but rather optimal oral health care must also incorporate the needs of the individual patient, as assessed by the attending dentist. More recently, the ADA established the Center for Evidence-Based Dentistry. The center's primary goals are to disseminate critically appraised information of current scientific evidence related to oral health and help dentists implement EBD in their practices.

It is well known that implementation of research evidence into clinical practice is an important component of any health care practice.[5–7] However, research findings are often inadequately disseminated and translated to practitioners, and practitioners tend to resist applying new information.[8] Numerous barriers stand in the way of translation and dissemination of evidence, two of which are limited access to scientific information and lack of time to identify, critically assess, and implement evidence.[9–16]

Since the inception of EBM in the early 1990s, the rapid growth of the Internet has made it easier for practitioners to gain access to the most current evidence. Use of computer-based systems for information retrieval has had an important impact on health care.[15] These kinds of advances in technology, because they offer the potential of delivering real-time information at the point of care, have a role helping to overcome the barriers of access to information and time constraints. Multiple online resources are available to dental professionals. These are cited elsewhere.[17,18] Examples of

> **Box 2**
> **The ADA definition of EBD**
>
> Evidence-based dentistry (EBD) is an approach to oral health care that requires the judicious integration of systematic assessments of clinically relevant scientific evidence, relating to the patient's oral and medical condition and history, with the dentist's clinical expertise and the patient's treatment needs and preferences.
>
> *Data from* American Dental Association, ADA policy on evidence-based dentistry. Available at: http://ada.org/prof/resources/positions/statements/evidencebased/asp. Accessed June 16, 2008.

such resources include Web sites with summaries of systematic reviews (**Table 1**) and Web sites for identifying evidence-based clinical recommendations or guidelines (**Table 2**).

As EBD continues to evolve, it is expected that implementation by practitioners will occur gradually as well. The diffusion of innovation theory describes the different stages of adopting new ideas, technologies, or methods.[19] This theory proposes that a limited number of individuals—the innovators and early adopters—are the first to take hold of new concepts. These innovators and early adopters influence the remainder of the population. Anecdotal information suggests that this theory holds for EBD; groups of innovators and early adopters first implemented EBD and influenced other dentists.[20]

In partnership with the *Journal of Evidence-Based Dental Practice* and supported by an educational grant from Procter & Gamble, the ADA established the EBD Champion program to leverage the knowledge, experience, and influence of those currently implementing EBD, the innovators and early adopters.[20,21] This program will develop a network of oral health care workers who will assist their colleagues to implement evidence-based approaches to practice. As part of an ongoing program, practitioners throughout the United States are recruited to become EBD Champions. These individuals learn how to implement EBD using a number of resources currently available and to ultimately disseminate their learning and experience to colleagues. Thus, the EBD Champions serve as a resource to the practitioners in their communities.

It is clear that dentists, members of the dental team, and patients are the primary targets for the continued evolution of EBD. However, this evolution has also revealed many other stakeholders with integral roles in EBD. We have discussed above the role of professional associations, specifically the ADA, but other stakeholders include policy makers, third-party payers, the dental industry, and educators.

EVIDENCE-BASED DENTISTRY AND DENTAL EDUCATION

Contemporary dental education in the United States is the result of several hundred years of educational evolution and innovation. The self-training and apprenticeship-training approaches, common up through the early 19th century, began to end with the opening of the first United States dental school, in Baltimore in 1840, and the first university-based dental department, at Harvard in 1867.[22] Although change occurred

Table 1
Online summaries of systematic reviews

Resource	Link
ADA	http://www.ada.org/goto/ebd
Database of Abstracts of Reviews of Effectiveness	http://www.crd.york.ac.uk/CRDWeb/
National Library for Health—Oral Health Specialist Library	http://www.library.nhs.uk/oralhealth/
Evidentista (Pan American Centers for Evidence-Based Dentistry)	http://us.evidentista.org/?o=1026
Bandolier: Dental and Oral Health	http://www.jr2.ox.ac.uk/bandolier/booth/booths/dental.html
Cochrane Oral Health Group	http://www.ohg.cochrane.org/reviews.html
Centre for Evidence-Based Dentistry	http://www.cebd.org/?o=1069

| Table 2 | |
| Online clinical recommendations/guidelines | |
Resource	Link
National Guideline Clearinghouse	http://www.guidelines.gov
ADA Evidence-Based Clinical Recommendations	http://www.ada.org/prof/resources/ebd/clinical.asp
PubMed Clinical Queries (National Library of Medicine)	http://www.ncbi.nlm.nih.gov/entrez/query/static/clinical.shtml#reviews
National Institute for Health and Clinical Excellence	http://www.nice.org.uk/guidance/index.jsp?action=byTopic&o=7298&set=true

slowly, an early watershed event in dental education was the release of the Gies Report in 1926,[23] which resulted in the closing of many proprietary dental schools and the eventual mandate that all dental schools be university-based and operate under an accreditation process to ensure educational quality and consistency.

Once dental education became universally housed within universities, steady progress toward a science-based curriculum became evident. Concomitant with this was the development of the concept of professionalism and the perceived need for standards of practice and ethical guidelines. As a result, dentistry began to take on more of the look of a medical subspecialty, with dental education paralleling many of the educational changes occurring in medicine.

In the latter part of the 20th century, due to the parallel development of clinical epidemiology and evidence-based medicine, there was a call for changes in medical education and clinical practice. Teaching the principles of evidence-based medicine during medical education was seen as an important component of the broader changes to medical practice that were needed. These changes occurred rapidly and, by the end of the 1990s, nearly 90% of United States medical schools offered EBM courses.[24]

Dentistry found itself similarly afflicted by wide variations in practice patterns and continued use of outdated approaches to treatment. In reviews of dental education, both the Institute of Medicine[22] and the Santa Fe Group[25] indicted the dental school curriculum as contributing to the problem and both called for substantial reforms. These reforms included a significant increase in curriculum time devoted to teaching the principles of EBD.

The degree to which dental schools have incorporated these recommended changes is not well documented. However, it is unlikely that the proportion of United States dental schools devoting significant curriculum time to EBD is anywhere near the 100% rate now found in medical schools. The University of Kentucky's efforts to use evidence-based protocols as a foundation for clinical teaching are described elsewhere in this issue.

Pressure to improve the teaching of EBD will continue in dentistry as the need for effective and efficient dental care continues to grow. Fortunately, awareness of the importance of EBD is now increasing through the efforts of the ADA and the American Dental Education Association. The legitimacy and visibility provided to EBD by the activities of organized dentistry will ultimately lead to greater participation by practicing dentists and dental schools. Many believe that universal teaching of EBD in dental school will only be assured, however, by the incorporation of EBD into accreditation guidelines.

Introducing EBD concepts at the level of first professional dental education is perhaps the most efficient and effective means of increasing its use in private practice.

However, it will take many years for this approach alone to diffuse into the profession. If we hope to see important changes in professional behavior within a reasonable time period, efforts must be made to increase EBD competency within the existing practicing community. We realize that, as with any significant change in the approach to practice, efforts to promote change will meet with resistance as it runs into well-established behaviors and attitudes set over years of practice. Nevertheless, we believe that the benefits of developing an evidence-based approach to care are well worth the effort. Moreover, when the full extent of these benefits are realized and the relative ease with which EBD can be incorporated into daily practice is understood, we feel that many dentists will embrace the concept and readily move into the next phase of dentistry. To that end, we provide below some of the benefits that can be derived from incorporating evidence-based thinking into the dental office.

BENEFITS FOR THE PRACTICING DENTIST

There are many potential benefits to dentists who use EBD in clinical practice. The most obvious and best reason is the prospect of obtaining improved patient health outcomes. Certainly this invokes our duties under the Hippocratic oath to "first do no harm" and, concomitantly, to provide the very best health care so patients may achieve and maintain optimum health. Other advantages dentists may garner include:

- Improved patient, staff, and dentist satisfaction
- Greater pride among patients, staff, and dentists in high-quality care
- Improved clinical decision-making capability[26]
- Greater confidence in treatment planning[26]
- More opportunity to provide treatment choices selected for minimizing risks of harm and maximizing treatment safety[26]
- Greater satisfaction derived from creating customized treatment plans based on the powerful combination of stronger scientific evidence, clinician judgment, and experience, as well as patient preferences and values[26]
- Increased day-to-day enjoyment working with a happier team motivated by working to a higher standard that puts the patient first in the dental care process[26]
- Reduced overhead and improved production by saving time and money using techniques and materials that are effective and efficient
- Higher treatment-plan acceptance as dentists add to their presentation tool box the sharing of high-quality meaningful evidence with patients
- Enhanced patient trust and rapport when patients who know their dentist relies on the highest level of evidence for making treatment recommendations
- Improved practice building opportunities as patients share with others their trust, confidence, and pride in their EBD-practicing dentist

Staff who are employed by EBD-practicing dentists also harvest many benefits, including:

- Increased staff confidence, pride, trust, and personal satisfaction[26]
- Enhanced recognition in the community and with peers as a thought-leader practice[26]
- Increased engagement and satisfaction in work when taught how to conduct EBD searches themselves, thereby directly contributing to the health of patients

Additionally and most importantly patients receive many benefits from EBD as well, including:

- Saved time and resources by choosing treatments that are more effective and efficient
- Customized treatment plans based upon the highest level of evidence, the lowest risk of harm, and the patient's personal preferences and needs
- Increased trust and confidence in the doctor and his or her practice[26]
- Greater incentive to invest in quality oral health care[26]
- Increased pride from being a patient of a community thought leader and distinctive practice

Once practitioners have mastered how and where to find EBD resources, they are ready for the next phase: prioritize clinical topics, organize the information found, and share the information with staff. There are many ways for dentists to prioritize the order of their searches. These include:

- According to diagnoses or interventions commonly found in the practice
- According to gaps in knowledge
- According to questions commonly asked by patients
- According to the procedure, treatment, or device considered for purchase or introduction into the practice

Each of these approaches is appropriate and the dentist may want to start with one topic per week and slowly begin to integrate the new knowledge into clinical practice. Information resulting from searches can be organized several ways, including on a computer in the office accessible to all staff (in a document or desktop folder or through the use of Microsoft OneNote), or printed and kept in a three-ring binder in the office and made accessible to all staff.

Clinicians may be uncomfortable at first with the tasks of introducing EBD concepts to staff and recommending appropriate changes according to the level of evidence. Staff and dentist alike can become very invested in a treatment philosophy, protocol, or procedure and, after reviewing evidence, a dentist may find information contrary to these ideas. The dentist must clearly define and voice to the staff from the beginning the practice's overall commitment to providing the very best patient care and the need to have the humility and open-mindedness to fulfill that commitment. Additionally, it is important to educate staff that EBD support is only part of the clinical decision-making process. Equally important factors are clinical experience and patient desires and needs. All data collected by EBD searches should be made easily accessible to staff. Regular staff meetings are the perfect opportunity to help explain EBD concepts, teach EBD searching techniques, and discuss levels of evidence found during recent searches. Staff can take great pride in knowing that they are providing the highest level of care. Proud, informed, and engaged staffmembers are likely to transmit this excitement to patients.

STRATEGIES FOR IMPLEMENTING EVIDENCE-BASED DENTISTRY
Preparing for Change

As with any change in clinical practice, the move to incorporate EBD involves more than just a desire to change. An attempt to change should first involve an analysis to identify factors likely to influence the proposed change.[27] If a clinician is to be successful in incorporating EBD in practice, reflection on current practice will be helpful. It is also worthwhile to identify both advantages for change and potential barriers to change.[28]

One systematic way to evaluate the potential for change is through a PESTLE analysis of strategic planning, which includes political, economic, social, technological, legal, and environmental (or ethical) factors.[29]

- Political influences include the positive momentum now evident through the efforts of the ADA and most specialist organizations. These political forces are quickly energizing clinicians to overcome the lukewarm response shown early in the EBD era.
- Economic factors are always a consideration in private as well as public dental models. Treatment based on the best evidence would seem to be more economical, but this remains to be shown. On the other hand, the old perception that EBD will reduce practice revenues is quickly giving way to the realization that adopting EBD is a practice-building move in the information age. Investments in training are expected with the adoption of any new technology, but the need for a computer and Internet access can hardly be considered unique to EBD. The decision to subscribe to library services or additional journals could represent financial investments.
- Social considerations may not be as obvious to dentists looking at EBD for the first time. The traditional culture of dentistry has been dominated by the pursuit of clinical competency. Evidence-based dentistry's additional emphasis on keeping up-to-date with research and critical thinking represents a paradigm shift for the profession.
- Technological issues in EBD include the skills of efficient searching, critically appraising, and regularly applying evidence in daily practice. Learning these skills represents a challenge. However, many dentists already have the foundation for these skills through the use of computers in many aspects of practice. Meanwhile, the science background intrinsic to dental education means that dentists tend to be comfortable with technical issues, which favors adoption of EBD.
- The legal aspect of adopting the EBD practice model includes risk reduction. When dentists use current research-based information in clinical decision-making, they diminish litigation risk. Including journal references in clinic notes provides verifiable support for clinical decisions.
- Ethical principles always take into account what is best for the patient. In EBD, the added dimension of using the best science supplements, but does not replace, the other skills of the treating dentist whose approach has always reflected the highest ethical standards.

Once the potential for change has been considered and a decision to adopt EBD has been made, a systematic approach to implementation is needed. Having a plan does not guarantee success, but the clinician without a plan for adoption is more likely to falter in the crucial first stages of implementation.

Implementing Evidence-Based Dentistry

When actually implementing EBD in practice, it may be useful to apply the SMART model. This acronym stands for specific, measurable, achievable (or agreed), realistic, and time bound.[30] As the EBD technique is adopted, it is useful to apply these attributes to the process.

When choosing a first subject, start with a clinical question you find interesting and that would yield benefits to a patient or group of patients. For example, the first goal could be to develop a policy for amalgam recommendations in the practice. The *specific* goal could be to write an office policy that conforms to the available evidence and is *measurable* in terms of adoption by the practice, *achievable* through application of the EBD methodology, *realistic* in answering specific questions about amalgam safety and effectiveness, and *time bound* in that a specific deadline is set for completion.

Continuing with our amalgam example, we next write a clinical question. This clinical question should be specific and include the appropriate structural elements, such as the PICO (patient [or problem], intervention, comparison, and outcome) format (**Table 3**).[31]

Of course, in developing a policy, more than one clinical question will be necessary. In the case of amalgam, other questions may address such factors as environmental impact, other safety issues, economic analysis, longevity, and postoperative complications.

Searching for Evidence

Set aside a time to complete your search. Allow at least 30 minutes for the first time a search is attempted. With practice, a much shorter search time will become possible.

Where to search is just as important as the clinical question. A Google search is a very common way to gather information, but the quality of the evidence is variable and the volume of sources or "hits" can be overwhelming. For example, typing in the search terms *children*, *amalgam*, *composite* from the above question into the Google search window will result in over 76,000 hits.

A more specific and judicious search can be achieved through PubMed or other search engines that access large bio-medical databases, such as Medline. Tutorials available on the PubMed Web site make it very user friendly. Other sources may be useful as well (see **Tables 1** and **2**).

Continuing with our example, a selective search of PubMed yielded several articles, including "Neurobehavioral Effects of Dental Amalgam in Children—A Randomized Clinical Trial" by DeRouen T, Matin M, Leroux B, and colleagues.[32] Once the search has yielded a body of evidence, it must be appraised. Of course evidence comes in many forms. In some sources, an additional layer of critical appraisal has been applied to research evidence. These sources include evidence-based clinical guidelines, systematic reviews, evidence summaries, and critical evaluations.

In other papers, the clinician must perform critical appraisal of original research results independently. These studies include randomized controlled trials (RCTs), cohort studies, case-control studies, and case reports. The research question and population or case in question determines the appropriateness of the study design. To aid in evaluating these papers, guides, such as the Critical Appraisal Skills Program (CASP) tools, are helpful. In our example, an appropriate tool would be "10 questions to help you make sense of randomized controlled trials."[33]

Table 3	
The PICO format for addressing clinical questions and an example of its application	
Question Element	**Example**
Patient or problem	In children with dental caries...
Intervention	Does placing amalgam restorations...
Comparison	Compared with composite restorations...
Outcome	Impact results of neurobehavioral assessments?

By applying the CASP tool or similar instruments, a stepwise approach to critical appraisal is more quickly and thoroughly accomplished. The CASP tool starts with two screening questions:

1. Did the study ask a clearly focused question in terms of the population studied, the intervention given, and the outcomes considered?

The answer to the first question is provided in the DeRouen article where the purpose is stated: "We report herein the results of a clinical trial comparing the health effects among children who had dental restoration performed using dental amalgam or resin composite materials." The paper also discussed the population, inclusion criteria, intervention, primary and secondary outcomes, measures of mercury exposure, health effects, and statistical analysis. We can answer the first question affirmatively.

2. Was this an RCT and was it appropriately so?

The DeRouen study met the criteria of an RCT. The strength of the interventional or therapeutic trial design and the prospective nature of the study lend credence to the appropriateness of the study in achieving the study goals. The answer to second question is yes.

At this point in the CASP tool, the decision to go on with the appraisal is made based on the answer to the first two screening questions. Because the paper showed strength in both questions, it is worthwhile to proceed with more in depth questions.

3. Were participants appropriately allocated to intervention and control groups?

Related in depth questions further aid the reviewer in answering this question. The article is explicit in describing the allocation of participants to the intervention and control groups and the characteristics of the groups' participants at the beginning of the trial are clearly delineated. It also clarifies how participants were assigned to the groups. The answer to the question is yes.

4. Were participants, staff, and study personnel "blind" to participants' study group?

The issue of blinding was addressed by the study. Participants could not be blinded to the intervention because of the obvious difference in appearance of the two restorative materials. Those measuring nerve conduction velocity (one of the primary outcomes of the study) were not aware of the group assignments. In this study, blinding of the participants is probably not an issue, so we can answer this question with a qualified yes.

5. Were all of the participants who entered the trial accounted for at its conclusion?

Once again the answer is yes. To account for all participants, the study went to great lengths, including an intention-to-treat analysis.

6. Were the participants in all groups followed up and data collected in the same way?

The answer appears to be yes. There were no apparent differences in interventions or testing applied to the two groups.

7. Did the study have enough participants to minimize the play of chance?

A power calculation was performed and sample sizes were determined prospectively. Also, an allowance was made for the predicted drop-out rate. For this question, the answer is yes.

8. How are the results presented and what is the main result?

The study showed no statistically significant differences in measures of memory, attention, visuomotor function, or nerve conduction rates for the amalgam and composite groups as reported by average z scores.

9. How precise are the results?

Univariate mean z scores and 95% confidence intervals were reported for each primary outcome.

10. Were all important outcomes considered so the results can be applied?

This question is open to interpretation by individual clinicians as the application of results depends on comparisons of the patient populations in the study and the individual practice respectively. In addition, there are numerous parameters of comparison that could be considered. On the other hand, the stated purpose of the study was met and it is unlikely that the patients in most practices would differ significantly from the population in the study.

The DeRouen study proved to be valid for most of the detailed questions from the CASP tool. Attention to detail in the design and execution of the study makes it a good example of an RCT.

Although the application of the CASP tool is a somewhat daunting task for the first-time appraiser, it allows a comprehensive and systematic approach to critical appraisal and expedites the procedure. As with any new skill, ease and speed are gained with repeated use.

As we develop a policy for amalgam recommendations in our practice, we can apply the evidence from the DeRouen article and feel confident that neurobehavioral effects of amalgam versus composite are insignificant in children up to 7 years after treatment.

Sometimes it is possible to complete searches in the operatory and present the results immediately to the patient. This has the advantage of being fast, and takes advantage of inquisitive momentum. At other times it may be prudent to complete the search and appraisal before sharing the evidence with the patient. This approach is useful with emerging issues in dentistry where more study and contemplation are called for.

It may be helpful to develop a script or outline when preparing to communicate evidence with patients. Of course we should also remember the difference between association and causation when epidemiologic studies are used. The script or outline can help organize our thoughts and aids in preparing a written summary of our discussion with the patient. The summary, including literature citations, can be stored in the chart as evidence of what was discussed.

There are several appropriate times for discussing evidence with patients. One excellent time is during patient education as part of hygiene appointments. Another time evidence can be helpful is while presenting fees and making payment arrangements when patients occasionally need to be reminded that treatment may be a good health care choice regardless of whether it is an insurance-covered benefit.

Dedicated treatment-planning appointments are an obvious time to discuss evidence with patients. This is especially true when the patient has misconceptions based on weak or faulty evidence. Patients generally consider the dentist and staff to be authoritative sources of information.[34] This fact alone should serve as an impetus to be a purveyor of the best evidence.

When EBD principles are applied, the patient-care decisions are ideally based on the best evidence available, the clinical skills and patient assessment by the dentist, and the patient's preferences and values.[35] It would be difficult to overestimate the value of this systematic, inclusive approach.

SUMMARY

Dentistry over the last 100 years has been characterized by improved approaches to education and practice. Parallel to trends in the field of medicine as a whole, dentistry is moving toward evidence-based practices. The goal of EBD is the assurance, through reference to high-quality evidence, that care provided is optimal for the patient and that treatment options are presented in a manner that allows for fully informed consent. As we transition toward broad-based use of EBD approaches in clinical practice, many dental offices will benefit from a better understanding of how EBD can improve patient outcomes. This article lists the likely benefits EBD can provide to patients, staff, and dentists when routinely adopted in daily practice.

Adopting EBD requires a willingness to be open to change as well as the skill needed to access high-quality evidence on optimal approaches to care. The ongoing growth of EBD resources on the Internet is making access to high-quality evidence uncomplicated and nearly effortless for almost any dental professional.

REFERENCES

1. Evidence-based medicine. A new approach to teaching the practice of medicine. JAMA 1992;268(17):2420–5.
2. Centre for evidence-based medicine. Available at: http://www.cebm.net/. Accessed June 16, 2008.
3. Sackett DL, Rosenberg WM, Gray JA, et al. Evidence based medicine: what it is and what it isn't. BMJ 1996;312(7023):71–2.
4. Sackett D, Straus SE, Richardson WS, et al. Evidence-based medicine: how to practice and teach EBM. 2nd edition. London: Churchill Livingtone; 2000.
5. Hunt DL, Haynes RB, Hanna SE, et al. Effects of computer-based clinical decision support systems on physician performance and patient outcomes: a systematic review. JAMA 1998;280(15):1339–46.
6. Balas EA, Austin SM, Mitchell JA, et al. The clinical value of computerized information services. A review of 98 randomized clinical trials. Arch Fam Med 1996; 5(5):271–8.
7. Anusavice KJ. Informatics systems to assess and apply clinical research on dental restorative materials. Adv Dent Res 2003;17:43–8.
8. Feifer C, Fifield J, Ornstein S, et al. From research to daily clinical practice: what are the challenges in "translation"? Jt Comm J Qual Saf 2004;30(5):235–45.
9. Koch S. Designing clinically useful systems: examples from medicine and dentistry. Adv Dent Res 2003;17:65–8.
10. Minton K. Perspective of a practicing dentist on the concept of evidence-based dentistry. Tex Dent J 2004;121(5):374–8.
11. Ismail AI, Bader JD. Evidence-based dentistry in clinical practice. J Am Dent Assoc 2004;135(1):78–83.
12. Iqbal A, Glenny AM. General dental practitioners' knowledge of and attitudes towards evidence based practice. Br Dent J 2002;193(10):587–91 [discussion: 83].
13. McKenna HP, Ashton S, Keeney S. Barriers to evidence-based practice in primary care. J Adv Nurs 2004;45(2):178–89.

14. Newman M, Papadopoulos I, Sigsworth J. Barriers to evidence-based practice. Intensive Crit Care Nurs 1998;14(5):231–8.

15. Hersh WR, Hickam DH. How well do physicians use electronic information retrieval systems? A framework for investigation and systematic review. JAMA 1998;280(15):1347–52.

16. Aurbach FE. Evidence-based dentistry: a practitioner's perspective. J Am Coll Dent 1999;66(1):17–20.

17. ADA.org. Evidence locator. Available at: http://www.ada.org/prof/resources/ebd/conferences_evidence.pdf. Accessed June 19, 2008.

18. Dentistry CfE-b. Dental Links. Available at: www.cebd.org/?o=1009. Accessed June 16, 2008.

19. Rogers E. Diffusion of innovations. New York: Free Press of Glencoe; 1962.

20. Frantsve-Hawley J, Meyer DM. The evidence-based dentistry champions: a grassroots approach to the implementation of EBD. J Evid Based Dent Pract 2008;8(2):64–9.

21. ADA.org. Evidence-based dentistry: Champion Conference. Available at: http://www.ada.org/prof/resources/ebd/conferences_champion.asp. Accessed June 16, 2008.

22. Committee on the Future of Dental Education. Institute of Medicine. Dental Education at the Crossroads Challenges and Change Committee on the Future of Dental Education. Marilyn J. Field, editor, Division of Health Care Services Institute of Medicine, National Academy Press, Washington, DC 1995.

23. Gies WJ. Dental education in the U.S. and Canada: a report to the Carnegie Foundation for the Advancement of Teaching. New York: Carnegie Foundation for the Advancement of Teaching; 1926.

24. Green ML. Graduate medical education training in clinical epidemiology, critical appraisal, and evidence-based medicine: a critical review of curricula. Acad Med 1999;74(6):686–94.

25. Dominick P, DePaola, Harold C. Reforming dental health professions education: a white paper. J Dent Educ 2004;68(11):1139–50.

26. The evidence-based dental (EBD) advantage. The American Dental Association. Available at: http://www.ada.org/prof/resources/ebd/conferences_practice.pdf. Accessed June 23, 2008.

27. NHS Centre for Reviews and Dissemination (1999) Effective health care-getting evidence into practice. Available at: http://www.york.ac.uk/inst/crd/. Accessed January 22, 2005.

28. Mind tools—essential tools for an excellent career, Force Field Analysis. Available at: http://www.mindtools.com/pages/article/newTED_06.htm. Accessed June 16, 2008.

29. Rapid BI, PEST/PESTLE analysis tool and template. Available at: http://www.rapidbi.com/created/the-PESTLE-analysis-tool.html. Accessed June 17, 2008.

30. The SMART Model on the Practice of Leadership Website. Available at: http://www.thepracticeofleadership.net/2006/03/11/setting-smart-objectives/. Accessed June 16, 2006.

31. Guyatt G, Drummond R. Users' guides to the medical literature—a manual for evidence-based clinical practice. JAMA & Archives Journals, American Medical Association: 2002. p. 16–20.

32. DeRouen T, Matin M, Leroux B, et al. Neurobehavioral effects of dental amalgam in children—a randomized clinical trial. JAMA 2006;295(15):1784–92.

33. Critical Appraisal Skills Program. Available at: www.phru.nhs.uk/Doc_Links/rct%20appraisal%20tool.pdf. Accessed June 17, 2008.

34. Chapple H, Shah S, Caress AL, et al. Exploring dental patients' preferred roles in treatment decision-making—a novel approach. Br Dent J 2003;194:321-7.
35. Needleman I. Introduction to evidence based dentistry. In: Clarkson J, Harrison J, Ismail A, Needleman I, Worthington H, editors. Evidence-based dentistry for effective practice. London: Martin Dunitz Publishing; 2003. p. 3.

In-Office Treatment of Dentinal Hypersensitivity

Mohanad Al-Sabbagh, DDS, MS[a],*, Amanda Brown[b],
Mark V. Thomas, DMD[c]

KEYWORDS

• Hypersensitivity • Dentinal • Tubules • Desensitize

Dentinal hypersensitivity (DH) is a common dental complaint in adults.[1–3] In most cases the pain response is initiated and persists only during the application of a suitable stimulus to the exposed dentin surface.[4] DH may occur when dentinal tubules are exposed to the oral environment due to recession and loss of tooth structure. DH is provoked when exposed dentin is subjected to stimuli such as osmotic changes, thermal changes, or mechanical stimuli such as toothbrushing. It has been suggested that DH is mediated by a hydrodynamic mechanism in which a stimulus results in increased fluid flow in the dentinal tubules.[3,5,6] This, in turn, activates nerves located on the pulpal aspect of the tubules, resulting in the generation of action potentials which are interpreted as pain by the patient.

There is some controversy regarding exactly what constitutes DH. For example, the European Federation of Periodontology uses the term "root sensitivity" (RS) to describe the DH-like sensitivity seen as a result of periodontal disease or treatment. It is conceivable that there may be a difference between long-standing DH in a patient with incipient recession and very good hygiene and that RS seen in a periodontal patient immediately following flap surgery.

Loss of enamel or cementum (and periodontal tissues) may result in exposed dentin. In 5% to 10% of teeth, the cementum does not reach the cementoenamel junction (CEJ) resulting in exposed dentin.[7] Loss of enamel or tooth structure occurs by attrition, abrasion, or erosion; whereas denudation of the root surface can occur as a result of gingival recession, periodontal therapy, or improper tooth brushing.[8–12] It has been reported that scaling and root planing may cause increased DH.[13] This is probably

[a] Division of Periodontology, University of Kentucky College of Dentistry, 800 Rose Street, Room D-438, Lexington, KY 40536-0297, USA
[b] Division of Periodontology, University of Kentucky College of Dentistry, 800 Rose Street, Room M-122, Lexington, KY 40536-0297, USA
[c] Department of Oral Health Practice, Division of Periodontology, University of Kentucky College of Dentistry, 800 Rose Street, Room M-122, Lexington, KY 40536-0297, USA
* Corresponding author.
E-mail address: malsa2@email.uky.edu (M. Al-Sabbagh).

Dent Clin N Am 53 (2009) 47–60
doi:10.1016/j.cden.2008.11.003
0011-8532/08/$ – see front matter. Published by Elsevier Inc.

dental.theclinics.com

because scaling and root planing (and periodontal surgical procedures) may remove the thin outer layer of cementum in the cervical third of the root, thus exposing the dentinal tubules.[14] Gillam and colleagues[15] reported that a significant number of patients reported DH following restorative treatment, but this study used a survey technique and it is possible that some patients may have actually been reporting hypersensitivity from microleakage or operative trauma.

DH is more accurately described as a symptom rather than a true disease entity. It is characterized as transient sharp pain originating from various types of stimuli. A number of other dental conditions such as carious lesions, cracked tooth syndrome, fractured restorations or teeth, periodontal disease, postoperative hypersensitivity, palatal-gingival grooves, enamel defects, a congenitally open CEJ, improperly insulated metallic restorations, occlusal traumatism, and tooth whitening may produce similar symptoms.[14] According to a recent review, "DH is usually diagnosed after other possible conditions have been eliminated" and may be considered a diagnosis of exclusion.[3] The role of plaque as an etiologic factor in DH is not resolved, although it has been suggested that dental plaque promotes and sustains DH, and that plaque control is important in preventing its development.[16] However, it has been noted that hypersensitive dentin is often found in toothbrush abrasion areas that are almost plaque-free.[14,17,18] Suge and colleagues[19] recently demonstrated in a dog model that the patency of dentinal tubules was more reduced in teeth subjected to stringent plaque control. These authors suggest that plaque control may promote the natural resolution of DH in some circumstances.

The prevalence of DH in the adult population ranges between 8% and 35%.[20,21] It has been reported that DH affects about 40 million adults in the United States.[22] In an international survey, Murray and Roberts[23] found that the prevalence of hypersensitive teeth was consistent across all the countries surveyed, affecting approximately 15% of the population. It has been shown that there is a slightly higher predilection of DH in females than males.[15,24,25]

The peak prevalence of DH has been variously reported as occurring between the second and fifth decades of life. Orchardson and Collins[24] reported a peak between 20 and 25 years, whereas Addy[21,26] found peak prevalence to occur at the end of the third decade. Fischer and colleagues[27] found it to be between 40 and 49 years.

DH most commonly occurs on the buccal aspect of permanent teeth near the CEJ, which is also the site that most frequently exhibits dentin exposure.[17,25] Dentin exposure may also occur on occlusal and lingual cervical surfaces, but hypersensitivity is rarely reported in these locations. With regard to tooth type, it has been reported that canines and premolars in either arch are the most frequently involved.[17,24,28]

Although DH can be very troubling to some patients, Gillam and colleagues[21,29] found that most individuals affected with DH did not perceive it to be a severe problem and consequently did not seek treatment. For example, only one in four patients with DH reported use of a desensitizing toothpaste.

Several factors can reduce dentin permeability and subsequently contribute to the spontaneous remission of DH. For example, a dentin smear layer often covers the exposed surface of dentin and may occlude the dentinal tubules, thereby reducing DH.[30] Adherence of salivary proteins to the dentinal surface and adherence of plasma proteins to the inner dentin surface may also reduce hypersensitivity, as can the formation of less permeable reparative dentin by the pulp.[31,32] Finally, the obturation of tubules by the formation of intratubular crystals from salivary minerals, dentinal fluids' mineral deposits, and calculus formation on the surface of dentin all reduce permeability.[6]

These natural mechanisms can be used to explain the clinical course of DH following periodontal surgery. During root planing, tubules remain occluded by the smear layer created by root surface debridement. This smear layer may reduce permeability and also lowers hydraulic conductance by blocking fluid movement.[30] As the smear layer dissolves, however, the permeability of dentin increases, resulting in the symptoms of DH in some patients. This occurs about 1 week after periodontal surgery, correlating with the observation of subjects having the highest DH rates 1 to 3 weeks postoperatively. Within a few weeks, the tubules may become partially occluded (eg, with crystalline deposits), thus decreasing permeability to bacterial products and intraoral stimuli.[30] This correlates with the decreased DH symptoms within a period of 6 weeks postsurgery.

DH affects as many as 40 million adults in the United States.[22] It is likely that the incidence of DH will increase because people are retaining their teeth longer, are living longer, and more dental root surfaces are exposed through gingival recession, scaling and root planing, and periodontal surgery.[33] Therefore, identifying its mechanisms and causes may become more important.

SPONTANEOUS RESOLUTION OF DENTINAL HYPERSENSITIVITY

Several factors can reduce dentin permeability and may contribute to the spontaneous remission of DH. There are a variety of mechanisms by which natural obturation of permeable tubules can occur. As noted above, formation of a smear layer covers exposed dentinal surfaces and may occlude dentinal tubules.[34] Dentin covered with a smear layer may be less hypersensitive, although this is a difficult concept to test experimentally.[30] In any event, the smear layer is easily removed and is, therefore, unlikely to provide any meaningful protection against DH.

Dental professionals have a variety of interventions to manage DH, including in-office treatments and self-applied products for home use. Much of the literature on the treatment of DH is anecdotal. There are few well-powered clinical trials that have examined interventions for DH. The purpose of this review is to review and critique the various treatment modalities for DH.

SEARCH STRATEGY

The search mechanism for this review included a MEDLINE search to identify English-language articles published between 1960 to 2007. The following search terms, including terms truncated with an asterisk, were used:

    dentinal
    dentin*
    hypersensitivity
    hypersensitiv*
    sensitivity
    desensiti*
    desensitiz*
    oxalate*
    resin*
    laser*

Various combinations of these terms were used. The "related articles" feature of PubMed was also used to identify additional citations. The searches yielded a large number of citations, most of which were found to represent a low level of evidence (eg, small exploratory studies and in vitro experiments). All returned citations were examined by title and abstract to ascertain applicability. The original inclusion criteria were human studies of these types: randomized clinical trials, clinical trials, meta-analyses, systematic reviews, or evidence-based practice guidelines. If the content was related to the research question and met the criteria, then the full report was retrieved. Very few publications met even the most liberal interpretation of the inclusion criteria.

A more focused search was then conducted, using the search terms "dentinal hypersensitivity" and using the "limits" tool to restrict the search to clinical trials, meta-analyses, practice guidelines, and randomized controlled trials. This search was also limited to English-language publications. Twenty-five citations were returned, of which none were systematic reviews of the topic. Only seven of the reports were published since 2000. Most were small pilot or exploratory studies that tested only two interventions.[35] The more inclusive search did yield a number of narrative reviews, but none were systematic reviews or meta-analyses.[3,12,36,37] Thus, the level of evidence in support of any intervention is rather weak, according to the techniques of evidence-based health care.[38,39] The remainder of this article describes and analyzes the results of this search as it applies to in-office interventions for DH. However, the level of evidence is insufficient to permit definitive recommendations regarding the management of this condition. Owing to the paucity of high-level evidence, a systematic review of this topic is not possible at this time. Therefore, this article has, of necessity, been configured as a narrative review.

CLINICAL MANAGEMENT OF DENTINAL HYPERSENSITIVITY: IN-OFFICE TREATMENTS

Treatment of DH can be accomplished by covering the exposed tubules with soft tissue grafts or restorative materials, occluding the tubules with materials that cause precipitation of crystals within the tubules, desensitization by way of laser treatment, or through desensitization of the nerve fibers with potassium nitrate.[37] All of these techniques have been used, but few have been subjected to rigorous testing for efficacy.

A recent consensus statement on DH by the Canadian Advisory Board on Dentin Hypersensitivity came to a similar conclusion after reviewing the state of the literature.[40] These authorities stated that "the need for consensus recommendations was made evident by the lack of clear and robust evidence in the dental literature." This advisory board went on to say that the "high prevalence of the condition, underdiagnosis and widespread availability of noninvasive, efficacious and inexpensive preventive treatment further underscored the need for direction." This board developed an algorithm for diagnosis and treatment that is consistent with the evidence (**Fig. 1**).

Cavity Varnishes

Brannstrom[41] suggested the application of cavity lining and varnishes under restorations, so that the smear layer plugging open tubules is retained. In a narrative review of DH interventions, Wycoff[42] recommended the use of a copal varnish, since covering exposed dentin with a thin film of varnish often renders it nonhypersensitive. For more sustained relief, a 2% sodium fluoride-containing varnish can be applied. The duration of effect of this varnish is usually 3 months. Further studies by Pashley and colleagues[43] evaluated a series of commercial cavity varnishes and bases for efficacy in reducing dentin permeability. They reported that all cavity varnishes tested decreased dentin permeability by 20% to 50%. Use of a 5% sodium fluoride varnish has been shown to form a protective layer of calcium fluoride that inhibits fluid flow within tubules, which has been suggested to be effective in the treatment of DH.[44]

Corona and colleagues[45] compared the galium-aluminium-arsenide laser and sodium fluoride varnish (Duraphat) in the treatment of DH. They found no statistically significant difference between fluoride varnish and laser.

In a controlled study, Mazor and colleagues[46] evaluated the effect of topical application of a sustained-release device in the form of a varnish containing strontium chloride on DH. They found that varnish containing strontium chloride showed a marked decrease in DH as compared with the placebo and untreated group.

Corticosteroids

It has been suggested that the application of anti-inflammatory drugs such as glucocorticoids to cavity preparations and exposed dentin may reduce DH by way of their effect on pain mediators. However, there is little experimental evidence to support or refute the use of such agents. In a double-blind study, Lawson and Huff[47] found that paramethasone had a significant desensitizing action. Furseth and Mjor[48] have reported complete obturation of dentinal tubules; hence, reduction of dentin permeability after an application of a corticosteroids preparation to exposed dentin. Mjor[49,50] reported less pulpal inflammation following restoration with a corticosteroid-containing cement than with amalgam in a nonhuman primate model. In summary, there is insufficient evidence to support or refute the use of corticosteroids in the treatment of DH.

Calcium Compounds

Calcium hydroxide [Ca $(OH)_2$] has been used many years for the treatment of DH, particularly after root planing. Ca $(OH)_2$ has little or no direct effect on dentin sensory nerve activity.[51] However, it is thought that it induces peritubular dentin mineralization and, subsequently, less hypersensitive dentin[49] Calcium compounds have compared favorably to other desensitizing agents in vitro. For example, Suge and colleagues[52] examined occlusion of dentinal tubules by scanning electron microscopy (SEM) and reported that calcium phosphate precipitation was more effective than potassium oxalate in occluding dentinal tubules.

Levin and colleagues[33] found that the application of Ca$(OH)_2$ paste to hypersensitive exposed dentin resulted in an immediate decrease of DH in over 90% of treated teeth. Jorkjend and Tronstad[53] applied a paste of Ca$(OH)_2$ to the exposed root surface following periodontal surgery. A thin layer of methacrylate and periodontal dressing where placed on top of the Ca$(OH)_2$. After removing the dressing 7 days later, they found that the teeth were no longer hypersensitive to cold, air, carbohydrates, toothbrushing, toothpicks, scaling or ultrasonic devices. Giniger and colleagues[54] also found that amorphous calcium added to a 16% carbamide peroxide-equivalent bleaching gel, significantly reduced DH.

Yates and colleagues[55] assessed the therapeutic effect of amorphous calcium phosphate in the treatment of DH in a split-mouth, randomized, placebo-controlled study, and reported no significant difference between the calcium phosphate group and the placebo group at the 84 day posttreatment follow-up.

Oxalates

Oxalate-containing products are a popular agent for in-office treatment of DH. Oxalate desensitizing agents are easy to apply, safe, relatively inexpensive, and well-tolerated by patients. It has also been shown that potassium oxalate has both dentinal tubule obturation properties and inhibitory effects caused by the potassium ions actions on nerve activity.[32] Oxalate ions react with calcium to form insoluble calcium oxalate crystals that bind tightly to dentin and obturate the dentinal tubules.[56] It has been shown that a 3% monohydrogen monopotassium oxalate releases a high concentration of calcium ions and accelerates crystal formation.

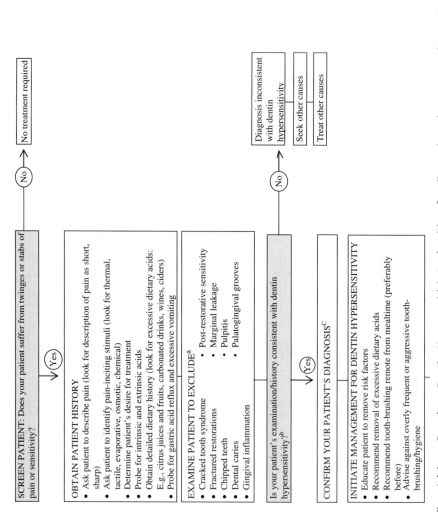

Fig. 1. Canadian Advisory Board on Dentin Hypersensitivity's algorithm for diagnosis and treatment. (*From* Canadian Advisory Board on Dentin Hypersensitivity. Consensus-based recommendations for the diagnosis and management of dentin hypersensitivity. J Can Dent Assoc 2003;69:222; with permission from the Canadian Dental Association.)

SCREEN PATIENT: Does your patient suffer from twinges or stabs of pain or sensitivity?

No → No treatment required

Yes

OBTAIN PATIENT HISTORY
- Ask patient to describe pain (look for description of pain as short, sharp)
- Ask patient to identify pain-inciting stimuli (look for thermal, tactile, evaporative, osmotic, chemical)
- Determine patient's desire for treatment
- Probe for intrinsic and extrinsic acids
- Obtain detailed dietary history (look for excessive dietary acids: E.g., citrus juices and fruits, carbonated drinks, wines, ciders)
- Probe for gastric acid reflux and excessive vomiting

EXAMINE PATIENT TO EXCLUDE[a]
- Cracked tooth syndrome
- Fractured restorations
- Chipped teeth
- Dental caries
- Gingival inflammation
- Post-restorative sensitivity
- Marginal leakage
- Pulpitis
- Palatogingival grooves

Is your patient's examination/history consistent with dentin hypersensitivity?[b]

No → Diagnosis inconsistent with dentin hypersensitivity → Seek other causes → Treat other causes

Yes

CONFIRM YOUR PATIENT'S DIAGNOSIS[c]

INITIATE MANAGEMENT FOR DENTIN HYPERSENSITIVITY
- Educate patient to remove risk factors
- Recommend removal of excessive dietary acids
- Recommend tooth-brushing remote from mealtime (preferably before)
- Advise against overly frequent or aggressive tooth-brushing/hygiene

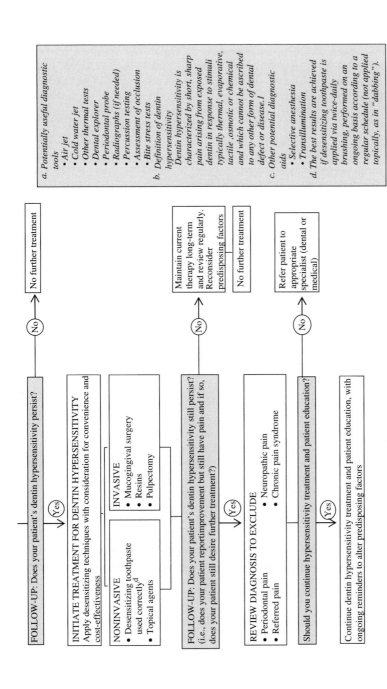

Fig. 1. (continued)

Three types of oxalates are available: 6% ferric oxalate, 30% dipotassium oxalate, and 3% monohydrogen monopotassium oxalate. In vitro studies have found that potassium oxalate preparations reduce dentin permeability.[57,58] There is evidence from animal studies that any relief provided may be relatively short-lived as the oxalate crystals are dissolved or removed over time.[59–61] Unfortunately, such in vitro and animal studies are, at best, suggestive and represent a weak level of evidence.

More relevant is an exploratory study by Pillon and colleagues[62] in which a single application of 3% potassium oxalate gel was applied following nonsurgical periodontal therapy. There was a significant reduction in DH on those teeth treated by 3% potassium oxalate compared with teeth treated with placebo. Unfortunately, the sample size was quite small (n = 15) and the duration of follow-up quite short (ie, 21 days posttreatment).

Oxalate-containing phytocomplexes have recently been investigated for possible effects on DH. For example, Sauro and colleagues[63] reported that dentinal permeability of extracted third molars was reduced after a single exposure to the oxalate-containing phytocomplexes. These same investigators have demonstrated that these phytocomplexes can protect the smear layer on recently instrumented dentin from removal by acidic soft drinks.[64] This finding may be worthy of additional research, as it has been shown that scaling and root planing produces a smear layer that reduces dentinal permeability, but this smear layer is acid-labile.[65]

While some of these reports are promising and worthy of further investigation, there is insufficient evidence to confirm the effectiveness of oxalates as an in-office treatment for DH.

Resins and Adhesives

The rationale for the use of resins and adhesives is to seal the dentinal tubules and hence to preclude the transmission of pain causing stimuli to the pulpal nerve fibers.[6] This mode of treatment is performed on localized hypersensitive dentin after other forms of treatment have failed. Resin-based materials have been reported to successfully reduce DH.[66,67] Unfortunately, many of the reports on these materials are in vitro studies which examine surrogate outcomes such as dentinal permeability.[68]

Brannstrom and colleagues[6] found that impregnating the dentinal tubules with a restorative resin material resulted in significant relief from DH. Wycoff[42] suggested that adhesives be used for severe cases of DH that were unresponsive to other interventions. He specifically recommended the use of a glass ionomer cement, but the evidence supporting this recommendation is weak. Copeland[69] reported successful treatment of DH for up to 18 months in 89% of hypersensitive teeth treated by Scotchbond.

A combination product consisting of an aqueous solution of 5% glutaraldehyde and 35% hydroxyethyl methacrylate (Gluma Desensitizer) has been reported to be an effective desensitizing agent for up to 9 months.[67,70] The glutaraldehyde intrinsically blocks dentinal tubules counteracting the hydrodynamic mechanism that leads to DH. It should be noted that a significant placebo effect was seen with water, which yielded reductions in DH ranging from 5% to 27%.[67] A subsequent study found that a low-viscosity glass ionomer was more effective than the glutaraldehyde-resin product at 25 months posttreatment.[71] This was a small pilot study involving 14 subjects.

In another small exploratory study of eight patients, lanzano and colleagues[72] evaluated the effectiveness of a dentin primer (N-tolylglycine-glycidyl methacrylate and bisphenyl dimethacrylate) in the treatment of DH. These investigators reported that a single application of the primer was effective over the 9-month study period.

In summary, resin restorations have been used to cover areas of denuded dentin. This would seem to be a rational treatment strategy. As noted above, some investigators have reported significant success with such interventions, but most of these studies suffered from small sample size. It would also be helpful to have information on the longevity and safety of such treatments. Larger studies will be needed to validate these interventions.

Laser Treatment

There are a number of reports that suggest that laser treatment may be useful in the treatment of DH, although definitive trials are lacking.[73] A recent review of the literature by Kimura and colleagues[74] reported that effectiveness of laser treatment of DH ranged from 5% to 100%. However, these authors also reported that the laser was less effective in cases of severe DH.

Moritz and colleagues[75] examined the long-term effects of combined carbon dioxide (CO_2) laser treatment and fluoridation on DH. He found that 97% of laser group showed complete relief from DH compared with conventional fluoridation. Furthermore, SEM examination at 18 months posttreatment showed complete closure of dentinal tubules. These authors concluded that the CO_2 laser is an ideal desensitizer for DH. More recently, Slutzky-Goldberg and colleagues[76] have demonstrated that CO_2 laser treatment resulted in decreased permeability of dentinal tubules as shown by a dye penetration test.

Zhang and colleagues[77] studied the effect of irradiated teeth by CO_2 laser on the pulp and in the treatment of DH. He found that all patients were free of DH immediately following laser treatment. Over 3 months, the CO_2 laser treatment reduced DH to air stimulus by 50% without obvious loss of pulpal vitality.

Lan and Liu[78] reported that the neodymium: yttrium-aluminum-garnet (Nd:YAG) laser reduced DH to air by 65% and to tactile stimulation by 77%. In a subsequent publication, these authors reported that Nd:YAG laser irradiation at can be used to seal the exposed dentinal tubules and suggested that this may be the mechanism by which DH is affected.[79]

In a clinical and SEM study, Kumar and Mehta[80] found that Nd:YAG laser irradiation in combination with 5% sodium fluoride varnish has higher efficacy in the management of DH than either treatment alone. The SEM findings were a reduction in number or patency of tubules.

Not all studies have reported positive results. In a double-blind, controlled, split-mouth clinical trial, Lier and colleagues[81] evaluated the efficacy of a single Nd:YAG laser application on treatment of DH versus negative control. There was no difference between the Nd:YAG laser group and the placebo group at 16 weeks.

The combination of a dental laser with other modes of treatment for DH was an effective and lasting dentinal tubule obturation procedure. Lan and colleagues[82] used SEM to evaluate the combination effect of sodium fluoride and Nd:YAG laser irradiation on human dentinal tubules in vitro. They found that 90% of dentinal tubules were occluded when fluoride varnish was first applied to exposed dentin and then treated with a ND:YAG laser. Furthermore, the fluoride varnish within the dentinal tubules could not be removed by electric toothbrushing. Once again, this is an in vitro study using a surrogate variable, as opposed to a clinical trial.

A combination of dental laser with dentin bonding agents has been reported to be an efficient method for improving dentin bonding.[82,83] Theoretically, this combination could provide better and more lasting occlusion of the dentinal tubules, although robust evidence to support this assertion is lacking. Vlacic and colleagues[84,85] reported the utility of using a laser-activated fluoride therapy to protect enamel from erosive challenges that could cause dentin exposure and hypersensitivity. Unfortunately, these were also in vitro studies that have yet to be tested in the clinical setting.

Some of the clinical studies using various lasers for treatment of DH report very encouraging results. However, additional studies are needed to conclusively demonstrate the utility and safety of such interventions.

Gingival Augmentation

Gingival reconstructive surgical periodontal procedures, such as root coverage grafts, have been used to treat DH due to gingival recession.[86–92] Although many investigators have reported on the efficacy of various methods of soft tissue augmentation for root coverage, it was not possible to locate any studies which were designed to specifically test such grafting as a treatment for DH. A PubMed search was conducted using the search terms "hypersensitivity" and "graft.*" The search was limited to clinical trials, meta-analyses, practice guidelines, and randomized controlled trials. Two of the citations involved soft tissue augmentation of recession defects, but neither was tested as an intervention for the treatment of DH. Broader searches were conducted, and studies were located that discussed postoperative sensitivity as an undesirable outcome, but no study was located that tested the reduction of DH as a primary aim. Thus, as with other in-office treatments for DH, the evidence is insufficient to provide definitive guidelines for clinical decision-making.

DISCUSSION

While there has been much written on the subject of DH, there have been few robust studies that would permit the creation of evidence-based clinical guidelines. In light of this, the authors propose that practitioners suggest reversible interventions which are unlikely to cause harm for most cases. In intractable or severe cases, it may be necessary to consider more invasive treatments, such as gingival augmentation; however, there is comparatively little evidence to suggest the relative effectiveness of such approaches. Clearly, this is an area which would benefit from additional research.

SUMMARY

DH is a common dental complaint. While a variety of therapies have been proposed to treat this condition, there have been few controlled trials conducted that would permit evidence-based decision-making. Most of the studies have been exploratory in nature. Further research is needed in this area, so that clinicians may offer their patients treatments based on best evidence. Until such evidence is available, it seems prudent to employ methods of therapy that are least likely to cause harm and are reversible.

REFERENCES

1. Berman LH. Dentinal sensation and hypersensitivity. A review of mechanisms and treatment alternatives. J Periodontol 1985;56(4):216–22.
2. Gillam DG, Orchardson R. Advances in the treatment of root dentine sensitivity: mechanisms and treatment principles. Endodontic Topics 2006;13(1):13–33.
3. Orchardson R, Gillam DG. Managing dentin hypersensitivity. J Am Dent Assoc 2006;137(7):990–8, quiz 1028–9.
4. Addy M. Etiology and clinical implications of dentine hypersensitivity. Dent Clin North Am 1990;34(3).
5. Brannstrom M. The hydrodynamic theory of dentinal pain: sensation in preparations, caries, and the dentinal crack syndrome. J Endod 1986;12(10):453–7.

6. Brannstrom M, Johnson G, Nordenvall KJ. Transmission and control of dentinal pain: resin impregnation for the desensitization of dentin. J Am Dent Assoc 1979;99(4):612–8.

7. Scott JH, Symons NB. Introduction to dental anatomy. Edinburgh: Churchill Livingstone; 1974.

8. Knight T. Erosion-abrasion. J Dent Assoc S Afr 1969;24(10):310–6.

9. Litonjua LA, Andreana S, Bush PJ, et al. Tooth wear: attrition, erosion, and abrasion. Quintessence Int 2003;34(6):435–46.

10. Amin WM, Al-Omoush SA, Hattab FN. Oral health status of workers exposed to acid fumes in phosphate and battery industries in Jordan. Int Dent J 2001; 51(3):169–74.

11. Litonjua LA, Andreana S, Bush PJ, et al. Toothbrushing and gingival recession. Int Dent J 2003;53(2):67–72.

12. Bamise CT, Olusile AO, Oginni AO. An analysis of the etiological and predisposing factors related to dentin hypersensitivity. J Contemp Dent Pract 2008;9(5):52–9.

13. von Troil B, Needleman I, Sanz M. A systematic review of the prevalence of root sensitivity following periodontal therapy. J Clin Periodontol 2002;29(Suppl 3): 173–7 [discussion 195–6].

14. Al-Sabbagh M, Andreana S, Ciancio SG. Dentinal hypersensitivity: review of aetiology, differential diagnosis, prevalence, and mechanism. J Int Acad Periodontol 2004;6(1):8–12.

15. Gillam DG, Seo HS, Newman HN, et al. Comparison of dentine hypersensitivity in selected occidental and oriental populations. J Oral Rehabil 2001;28(1):20–5.

16. Tammaro S, Wennstrom JL, Bergenholtz G. Root-dentin sensitivity following non-surgical periodontal treatment. J Clin Periodontol 2000;27(9):690–7.

17. Addy M, Mostafa P, Newcombe RG. Dentine hypersensitivity: the distribution of recession, sensitivity and plaque. J Dent 1987;15:242–8.

18. Addy M, Pearce N. Aetiological, predisposing and environmental factors in dentine hypersensitivity. Arch Oral Biol 1994;39(Suppl):33S–8S.

19. Suge T, Kawasaki A, Ishikawa K, et al. Effects of plaque control on the patency of dentinal tubules: an in vivo study in beagle dogs. J Periodontol 2006;77(3):454–9.

20. Chabanski MB, Gillam DG, Bulam JS, et al. Prevalence of cervical dentine hypersensitivity in a population of patients referred to a specialist periodontology department. J Clin Periodontol 1996;23:989–92.

21. Gillam DG, Sco HS, Bulman JS, et al. Perception of dentine hypersensitivity in a general practice population. J Oral Rehabil 1999;26:710–4.

22. Kanapka JA. Over-the-counter dentifrice in the treatment of tooth hypersensitivity, review of clinical studies. Dent Clin North Am 1990;34:545–60.

23. Murray LE, Roberts AJ. The prevalence of self-reported hypersensitivity teeth. Arch Oral Biol 1994;39(Suppl):129.

24. Orchardson R, Collins WJ. Clinical features of "hypersensitive" (HS) dentine. J Dent Res 1984;63:521 (abstract No. 282).

25. Flynn J, Galloway R, Orchardson R. The incidence of hypersensitivity teeth in the West of Scotland. J Dent 1985;13:230–6.

26. Addy M. Clinical aspects of dentin hypersensitivity. Proc Finn Dent Soc 1992; 88(Suppl 1):23–30.

27. Fischer C, Fischer RG, Wennberg A. Prevalence and distribution of cervical dentine hypersensitivity in a population in Rio de Janeiro, Brazil. J Dent 1992;20(5): 272–6.

28. Orchardson R, Collins WJ. Clinical features of hypersensitive teeth. Braz Dent J 1987;162:253.

29. Irwin CR, McCusker P. Prevalence of dentine hypersensitivity in a general dental population. J Ir Dent Assoc 1997;43(1):7–9.
30. Pashley DH. Mechanism of dentin sensitivity. Dent Clin North Am 1990;34(3): 449–70.
31. Pashley DH, Nelson R, Kepler EE. The effects of plasma and salivary constituents on dentin permeability. J Dent Res 1982;61(8):978–81.
32. Pashley DH. Dentin permeability, dentin sensitivity, and treatment through tubule occlusion. J Endod 1986;12:465–74.
33. Levin MP, Yearwood LL, Carpenter WN. The desensitizing effect of calcium hydroxide and magnesium hydroxide on hypersensitive dentin. Oral Surg Oral Med Oral Pathol 1973;35(5):741–6.
34. Greenhill JD, Pashley DH. The effects of desensitizing agents on the hydraulic conductance of human dentin in vitro. J Dent Res 1981;60(3):686–98.
35. Hujoel PP. Definitive vs. exploratory periodontal trials: a survey of published studies. J Dent Res 1995;74(8):1453–8.
36. Walters PA. Dentinal hypersensitivity: a review. J Contemp Dent Pract 2005;6(2): 107–17.
37. Jacobsen PL, Bruce G. Clinical dentin hypersensitivity: understanding the causes and prescribing a treatment. J Contemp Dent Pract 2001;2(1):1–12.
38. Guyatt G, Jaeschke R, Meade MO. Why study results mislead: bias and random error. In: Guyatt G, Rennie D, Meade MO, et al, editors. Users' guides to the medical literature: a manual for evidence-based clinical practice. New York: McGraw-Hill Medical; 2008. p. 59–66.
39. Guyatt G, Jaeschke R, Prasad K, et al. Summarizing the evidence. In: Guyatt G, Rennie D, Meade MO, et al, editors. Users' guides to the medical literature. New York: McGraw-Hill Medical; 2008. p. 523–54.
40. Consensus-based recommendations for the diagnosis and management of dentin hypersensitivity. J Can Dent Assoc 2003;69(4):221–6.
41. Brannstrom M. The cause of postrestorative sensitivity and its prevention. J Endod 1986;12(10):475–81.
42. Wycoff SJ. Current treatment for dentinal hypersensitivity. In-office treatment. Compend Contin Educ Dent 1982;(Suppl 3):S113–5.
43. Pashley DH, O'Meara JA, Williams EC, et al. Dentin permeability: effects of cavity varnishes and bases. J Prosthet Dent 1985;53(4):511–6.
44. Gaffar A. Treating hypersensitivity with fluoride varnish. Compend Contin Educ Dent 1999;20(1 Suppl):27–33, quiz, 35.
45. Corona SA, Nascimento TN, Catirse AB, et al. Clinical evaluation of low-level laser therapy and fluoride varnish for treating cervical dentinal hypersensitivity. J Oral Rehabil 2003;30(12):1183–9.
46. Mazor Z, Brayer L, Friedman M, et al. Topical varnish containing strontium in a sustained-release device as treatment for dentin hypersensitivity. Clin Prev Dent 1991;13(3):21–5.
47. Lawson BF, Huff TW. Desensitization of teeth with a topically applied glucocorticoid drug. A preliminary study. J Oral Ther Pharmacol 1966;2(4):295–9.
48. Furseth R, Mjor IA. The fine structure of corticosteroid-covered, human dentine. Arch Oral Biol 1972;17(4):719–28.
49. Mjor IA. Histologic studies of human coronal dentine following the insertion of various materials in experimentally prepared cavities. Arch Oral Biol 1967;12(4): 441–52.
50. Mjor IA, Lervik T. Pulp healing subjacent to corticosteroid-covered and amalgam-covered dentin. Oral Surg Oral Med Oral Pathol 1975;40(6):789–95.

51. Trowbridge H, Edwall L, Panopoulos P. Effect of zinc oxide-eugenol and calcium hydroxide on intradental nerve activity. J Endod 1982;8(9):403–6.
52. Suge T, Kawasaki A, Ishikawa K, et al. Comparison of the occluding ability of dentinal tubules with different morphology between calcium phosphate precipitation method and potassium oxalate treatment. Dent Mater J 2005;24(4):522–9.
53. Jorkjend L, Tronstad L. Treatment of hypersensitive root surfaces by calcium hydroxide. Scand J Dent Res 1972;80(3):264–6.
54. Giniger M, Macdonald J, Ziemba S, et al. The clinical performance of professionally dispensed bleaching gel with added amorphous calcium phosphate. J Am Dent Assoc 2005;136(3):383–92.
55. Yates R, Owens J, Jackson R, et al. A split-mouth placebo-controlled study to determine the effect of amorphous calcium phosphate in the treatment of dentine hypersensitivity. J Clin Periodontol 1998;25(8):687–92.
56. Trowbridge HO, Silver DR. A review of current approaches to in-office management of tooth hypersensitivity. Dent Clin North Am 1990;34(3):561–81.
57. Pashley DH, Leibach JG, Horner JA. The effects of burnishing NaF/kaolin/glycerin paste on dentin permeability. J Periodontol 1987;58(1):19–23.
58. Pashley DH, Carvalho RM, Pereira JC, et al. The use of oxalate to reduce dentin permeability under adhesive restorations. Am J Dent 2001;14(2):89–94.
59. Cooley RL, Sandoval VA. Effectiveness of potassium oxalate treatment on dentin hypersensitivity. Gen Dent 1989;37(4):330–3.
60. Knight NN, Lie T, Clark SM, et al. Hypersensitive dentin: testing of procedures for mechanical and chemical obliteration of dentinal tubuli. J Periodontol 1993;64(5):366–73.
61. Kerns DG, Scheidt MJ, Pashley DH, et al. Dentinal tubule occlusion and root hypersensitivity. J Periodontol 1991;62(7):421–8.
62. Pillon FL, Romani IG, Schmidt ER. Effect of a 3% potassium oxalate topical application on dentinal hypersensitivity after subgingival scaling and root planing. J Periodontol 2004;75(11):1461–4.
63. Sauro S, Gandolfi MG, Prati C, et al. Oxalate-containing phytocomplexes as dentine desensitisers: an in vitro study. Arch Oral Biol 2006;51(8):655–64.
64. Sauro S, Mannocci F, Watson TF, et al. The influence of soft acidic drinks in exposing dentinal tubules after non-surgical periodontal treatment: a SEM investigation on the protective effects of oxalate-containing phytocomplex. Med Oral Patol Oral Cir Bucal 2007;12(7):E542–8.
65. Fogel HM, Pashley DH. Effect of periodontal root planing on dentin permeability. J Clin Periodontol 1993;20(9):673–7.
66. Dondi dall'Orologio G, Lorenzi R, Anselmi M, et al. Dentin desensitizing effects of Gluma Alternate, Health-dent Desensitizer and Scotchbond Multi-Purpose. Am J Dent 1999;12(3):103–6.
67. Kakaboura A, Rahiotis C, Thomaidis S, et al. Clinical effectiveness of two agents on the treatment of tooth cervical hypersensitivity. Am J Dent 2005;18(4):291–5.
68. Tay FR, Gwinnett AJ, Pang KM, et al. Structural evidence of a sealed tissue interface with a total-etch wet-bonding technique in vivo. J Dent Res 1994;73(3):629–36.
69. Copeland JS. Simplified remedy for root sensitivity. Northwest Dent 1985;64(6):13–4.
70. Schupbach P, Lutz F, Finger WJ. Closing of dentinal tubules by Gluma Desensitizer. Eur J Oral Sci 1997;105(5 Pt 1):414–21.
71. Polderman RN, Frencken JE. Comparison between effectiveness of a low-viscosity glass ionomer and a resin-based glutaraldehyde containing primer in treating dentine hypersensitivity—a 25.2-month evaluation. J Dent 2007;35(2):144–9.

72. Ianzano JA, Gwinnett AJ, Westbay G. Polymeric sealing of dentinal tubules to control sensitivity: preliminary observations. Periodontal Clin Investig 1993; 15(1):13–6.
73. Cooper LF, Myers ML, Nelson DG, et al. Shear strength of composite bonded to laser-pretreated dentin. J Prosthet Dent 1988;60(1):45–9.
74. Kimura Y, Wilder-Smith P, Yonaga K, et al. Treatment of dentine hypersensitivity by lasers: a review. J Clin Periodontol 2000;27(10):715–21.
75. Moritz A, Schoop U, Goharkhay K, et al. Long-term effects of CO_2 laser irradiation on treatment of hypersensitive dental necks: results of an in vivo study. J Clin Laser Med Surg 1998;16(4):211–5.
76. Slutzky-Goldberg I, Nuni E, Nasralla W, et al. The effect of CO_2 laser on the permeability of dentinal tubules: a preliminary in vitro study. Photomed Laser Surg 2008;26(1):61–4.
77. Zhang C, Matsumoto K, Kimura Y, et al. Effects of CO_2 laser in treatment of cervical dentinal hypersensitivity. J Endod 1998;24(9):595–7.
78. Lan WH, Liu HC. Treatment of dentin hypersensitivity by Nd:YAG laser. J Clin Laser Med Surg 1996;14(2):89–92.
79. Lan WH, Lee BS, Liu HC, et al. Morphologic study of Nd:YAG laser usage in treatment of dentinal hypersensitivity. J Endod 2004;30(3):131–4.
80. Kumar NG, Mehta DS. Short-term assessment of the Nd:YAG laser with and without sodium fluoride varnish in the treatment of dentin hypersensitivity—a clinical and scanning electron microscopy study. J Periodontol 2005;76(7):1140–7.
81. Lier BB, Rosing CK, Aass AM, et al. Treatment of dentin hypersensitivity by Nd:YAG laser. J Clin Periodontol 2002;29(6):501–6.
82. Lan WH, Liu HC, Lin CP. The combined occluding effect of sodium fluoride varnish and Nd:YAG laser irradiation on human dentinal tubules. J Endod 1999; 25(6):424–6.
83. Dowell P, Addy M, Dummer P. Dentine hypersensitivity: aetiology, differential diagnosis and management. Braz Dent J 1985;158(3):92–6.
84. Vlacic J, Meyers IA, Kim J, et al. Laser-activated fluoride treatment of enamel against an artificial caries challenge: comparison of five wavelengths. Aust Dent J 2007;52(2):101–5.
85. Vlacic J, Meyers IA, Walsh LJ. Laser-activated fluoride treatment of enamel as prevention against erosion. Aust Dent J 2007;52(3):175–80.
86. Langer B, Langer L. Subepithelial connective tissue graft technique for root coverage. J Periodontol 1985;56(12):715–20.
87. Miller PD Jr. Root coverage using a free soft tissue autograft following citric acid application. Part 1: technique. Int J Periodontics Restorative Dent 1982;2(1):65–70.
88. Miller PD Jr. Root coverage using the free soft tissue autograft following citric acid application. II. Treatment of the carious root. Int J Periodontics Restorative Dent 1983;3(5):38–51.
89. Miller PD Jr. Root coverage using the free soft tissue autograft following citric acid application. Part III. A successful and predictable procedure in areas of deep-wide recession. Int J Periodontics Restorative Dent 1985;5(2):14–37.
90. Miller PD Jr. Root coverage with the free gingival graft. Factors associated with incomplete coverage. J Periodontol 1987;58(10):674–81.
91. Miller PD Jr. Using periodontal plastic surgery techniques. J Am Dent Assoc 1990;121(4):485–8.
92. Fombellida Cortazar F, Sanz Dominguez JR, Keogh TP, et al. A novel surgical approach to marginal soft tissue recessions: two-year results of 11 case studies. Pract Proced Aesthet Dent 2002;14(9):749–54, quiz 756.

Patient-Applied Treatment of Dentinal Hypersensitivity

Mohanad Al-Sabbagh, DDS, MS[a],*, Ershal Harrison, DMD[b],
Mark V. Thomas, DMD[c]

KEYWORDS

• Hypersensitivity • Dentinal • Desensitize

Dentinal hypersensitivity (DH) is defined as an exaggerated response to nonnoxious and noxious stimuli.[1] A more specific definition was provided by Holland and colleagues,[2] who stated that DH is a "short, sharp pain arising from exposed dentin in response to stimuli typically thermal, evaporative, tactile, osmotic, or chemical and which cannot be ascribed to another form of dental defect or pathology." The etiology and diagnosis of this condition is discussed by Sabbagh, Brown, and Thomas elsewhere in this issue. The purpose of this article is to examine the evidence regarding the effectiveness of various patient-applied interventions for DH.

TREATMENT OPTIONS FOR DENTINAL HYPERSENSITIVITY

A variety of patient-applied products have been developed for the treatment of DH.[3] The majority of products focus on blocking the mechanism of pain transmission, primarily by dentinal tubule obturation and increased pain threshold of sensory nerves. The goal of such therapies is to prevent the pain signal from being triggered. We will review the literature on various treatments for DH, both self-applied and in-office treatments.

Search Strategy

The search strategy for this review included a MEDLINE search (through PubMed) to identify English-language articles published between 1960 to 2007. The search terms used are shown in **Box 1**. Various combinations of these terms were used. The

[a] Division of Periodontology, University of Kentucky College of Dentistry, 800 Rose Street, Room D-438, Lexington, KY 40536-0297, USA
[b] Division of Comprehensive Care, University of Kentucky College of Dentistry, Lexington, KY 40536-0297, USA
[c] Department of Oral Health Practice, Division of Periodontology, University of Kentucky College of Dentistry, 800 Rose Street, Room M-122, Lexington, KY 40536-0297, USA
* Corresponding author.
E-mail address: malsa2@email.uky.edu (M. Al-Sabbagh).

Dent Clin N Am 53 (2009) 61–70
doi:10.1016/j.cden.2008.11.004
0011-8532/08/$ – see front matter. Published by Elsevier Inc.

<table>
<tr><td>

Box 1
Search terms used

dentin[a]

dentinal

desensiti[a]

desensitiz[a]

hypersensitiv[a]

hypersensitivity

laser[a]

oxalate[a]

resin[a]

sensitivity

strontium

[a] Commonly used conversions when researching electronic databases.

</td></tr>
</table>

"related articles" feature of PubMed was also used to identify additional citations. The searches yielded a large number of citations, most of which consisted of low-level evidence (eg, small exploratory studies and in vitro experiments). These reports were examined by title and abstract to ascertain relevance. If the content was related to the research question and met the original inclusion criteria (**Box 2**), then the full report was retrieved. Very few publications met even the most liberal interpretation of the inclusion criteria (see **Box 2**). The Cochrane Library was also searched for systematic reviews and reviews of effectiveness related to DH.

A more focused search was then conducted, using the search terms "dentinal hypersensitivity" and using the "limits" tool to restrict the search to clinical trials, meta-analyses, practice guidelines, and randomized controlled trials. This search was also limited to English-language publications. Twenty-five citations were returned, of which none were systematic reviews of the topic. Only seven of the reports had been published since 2000. Most were small pilot or exploratory studies that tested only two interventions.[4] The more inclusive search did yield a number of narrative reviews, but none were systematic reviews or meta-analyses.[4–8] Thus, the level of evidence in support of any intervention is rather weak, according to the techniques of evidence-based health care.[9,10] The remainder of this article describes and analyzes the results of this search as it applies to in-office interventions for DH, although it must be noted that the level of evidence is insufficient to permit definitive recommendations to be made regarding the management of this condition. Due to the paucity of high-level evidence,

<table>
<tr><td>

Box 2
Original inclusion criteria

Human studies

Study type: randomized clinical trials, clinical trials, meta-analyses, systematic reviews, or evidence-based practice guidelines

</td></tr>
</table>

this review has, of necessity, been configured as a narrative review, since a systematic review of this topic is not possible at this time.

Self-Applied Desensitizing Agents

The ideal patient-applied desensitizing agent should be nonirritating to the pulp, leave no deposits on tooth surfaces or restorations, and should not be irritating to the soft tissues. To ensure compliance the product should be easily applied, have a rapid onset, produce long-lasting relief, and provide effective relief from DH.

There are two major sites of action for self-applied DH-treatment products.[11] The majority of products reduce fluid movement through dentin by obturating the tubules. This concept is based on Brannstrom's hydrodynamic theory of DH which asserted that fluid movement in the dentinal tubules can generate action potentials in associated afferent nerve fibers. A second therapeutic strategy targets these nerve fibers. These products act to decrease the activity of dentinal sensory nerves thereby preventing the pain signal from being transmitted to the central nervous system. The mechanism of action for DH products can include one or both of these mechanisms. Many of these agents are reviewed below.

Strontium chloride

A PubMed search was conducted using the search term "strontium" in the title or abstract field (with limits set to dental journals only). Thirty-three citations were returned. Only three of these had been published since 2000. Strontium has been suggested to have several effects on teeth, including a cariostatic effect which is alleged to be most effective in the pre-eruptive phase of tooth formation.[12] Additionally, there is some evidence that strontium may have an effect on cariogenic bacteria when used topically.[13] Strontium can substitute for calcium in activating secretory mechanisms and can also possibly affect or modulate the pulpal cholinergic and adrenergic mechanisms involved in DH.[14]

The manner in which strontium affects DH has not been elucidated, but it has been proposed that the ions occlude dentinal tubules by binding to the tooth substance and stimulating reparative dentin formation. It has also been suggested that strontium ions have the capacity to reduce sensory nerve activity, but less effectively than potassium ions.[11] However, Kishore and colleagues[15] reported that strontium chloride is more effective than potassium nitrate. These workers demonstrated that 10% and 2% strontium chloride significantly reduced DH, while a 5% solution of potassium nitrate did not show a significant reduction in DH.

Dentifrices containing 10% strontium chloride have been widely used as desensitizing agents and were one of the first agents to be marketed for that purpose. Cohen found that 67% of the subjects using a strontium chloride-containing toothpaste reported complete relief of DH within a 2 month period.[16] Meffert and Hoskins[17] reported that 78% of the subjects achieved almost complete relief of DH. In a double-blinded, placebo-controlled study (n = 62), Minkoff and Axelrod[18] found that 10% strontium chloride is an effective treatment for DH. The effectiveness was evident within 2 weeks and lasted for the length of the 6-week study. Following periodontal surgery, Uchida and colleagues[19] treated DH patients with a 10% strontium chloride dentifrice. The 10% strontium chloride dentifrice was more effective in treating DH following periodontal surgery than a placebo dentifrice.

Some reports suggest that strontium is less effective than other desensitizing agents. For example, potassium nitrate has replaced strontium chloride in the treatment of DH. Silverman and colleagues[20] conducted a multicenter clinical trial that compared 5% potassium nitrate-containing dentifrices (with and without 0.243

percent sodium fluoride) with a 10% strontium chloride-containing dentifrice. The study sample consisted of 230 adults who were followed for 8 weeks. Both the potassium nitrate dentifrices were reported by subjects to be significantly superior to the negative placebo and strontium chloride dentifrices. Clinical evaluations gave similar results. The study was conducted in several private practices. This study was reasonably well-powered, but was of relatively brief duration. Other investigators have also reported the superiority potassium nitrate over strontium chloride.[21]

In summary, there is some evidence supporting the effectiveness of patient-applied strontium chloride as a treatment for DH, although the evidence is generally of low quality. One of the trials was a multicenter, placebo-controlled trial with a reasonable sample size. This study did demonstrate the superiority of two potassium nitrate toothpastes to a strontium chloride-containing dentifrice and a negative placebo.

Potassium

Potassium salts block neural transmission at the pulp and depolarize the nerve around the odontoblasts.[22] Potassium nitrate has been incorporated into both toothpastes and mouthrinses for use as a treatment for DH. Kim[23] reported for the first time that the potassium ion is the active portion of potassium nitrate. Greenhill and Pashley[24] found potassium nitrate ineffective in decreasing dentinal fluid flow in vitro coated dentin, even at 30% concentration. This suggests a lack of effect on fluid flow.

Products containing potassium have been studied to evaluate the efficacy of potassium nitrate as a desensitizing agent. For example, Tarbet and colleagues[25] found that a 5% potassium nitrate paste reduced DH effectively at 1 week and up to 4 weeks. Tarbet and colleagues[21] also compared the abilities of strontium chloride, dibasic sodium citrate, formaldehyde and potassium nitrate to desensitize hypersensitive teeth and reported that 5% potassium nitrate was the most effective in reducing DH.

More recently, Nagata and colleagues[26] compared the effectiveness of a 5% potassium nitrate dentifrice compared with placebo in a double-blind study and found a significant reduction in DH for subjects using potassium nitrate. Placebo subjects showed a 6% reduction in DH, while 67% of the potassium nitrate subjects reported complete relief throughout the 12 weeks of the study. As with many of the studies in this area, the sample size was small (N = 36).

Before the early 1990s, desensitizing dentifrices with potassium nitrate were not combined with fluoride agents in the United States. This was inconvenient, as many patients who wished to use the desensitizing dentifrices had to also use another toothpaste if they wished to receive the effect of the fluoride. In 1992, the US Food and Drug Administration considered the combination of 5% potassium nitrate and fluoride dentifrice as a safe and effective combined treatment option. In a multi-center double-blind controlled study, Silverman and colleagues[20] found that the combination of 5% potassium nitrate and 0.243% sodium fluoride in dentifrice is significantly more effective in the treatment of DH than a 10% strontium chloride-containing dentifrice. Additional clinical research has confirmed the effectiveness of the potassium nitrate–fluoride dentifrice in the treatment of DH.[27–31]

While most of the research in this area has used potassium nitrate, some investigators have used potassium citrate. Hu and colleagues[32] recently compared a dentifrice containing 5.5% potassium citrate to a commercially available dentifrice containing 3.75% potassium chloride, 0.32% sodium fluoride, and 0.3% triclosan in a silica base. There was no statistically significant difference between these formulations. This was an 8-week double-blinded study involving 80 subjects. Chesters and colleagues[33] compared a potassium citrate–sodium monofluorophosphate (PC–SMFP) dentifrice to potassium nitrate-SMFP and control dentifrices containing only SMFP and reported that the PC–SMFP was significantly more effective in reducing DH.

Whereas many studies have found potassium nitrate toothpastes to have some effect in reducing DH, a recent systematic review published in the Cochrane Database found "no clear evidence is available for the support of potassium-containing toothpastes for DH."[34]

Dibasic sodium citrate

In an in vitro study by Greenhill and Pashley,[24] a 19% reduction in dentinal fluid flow was thought to be attributable to dentinal tubule obturation. In a number of double-blind, placebo-controlled studies, dibasic sodium citrate was significantly superior to a placebo in reducing DH.[35–37] However, in a 6 week trial, sodium citrate dentifrice was not significantly more effective than a 0.76% SMFP control.

Fluoride-based interventions

Clinical trials have shown that some fluoride dentifrices or concentrated fluoride solutions are effective in producing favorable results in the treatment of DH.[38] Tal and colleagues[39] proposed that precipitated fluoride compounds may reduce DH by occlusion of the dentinal tubules. In a 3 month study, Kanouse and Ash[40] reported that subjects using a monofluorophosphate (MFP) dentifrice had a statistically significant increased tolerance to cold and hot in comparison to subjects using a placebo dentifrice.

Stannous fluoride has also been proposed as a treatment for DH. Thrash and colleagues[41] noted that topical application of 0.717% aqueous stannous fluoride (SnF_2) gave patients immediate relief from DH. Blong and colleagues[42] found that application of 0.4% SnF_2 gel was also an effective treatment for DH. However, prolonged use of the SnF2 gel with a minimum of 4 weeks of treatment was necessary to achieve satisfactory results.

Schiff and colleagues[43] recently examined the efficacy and safety of a toothpaste containing 0.454% stabilized SnF_2 and sodium hexametaphosphate (SHMP). The control dentifrice was a sodium fluoride dentifrice. The double-blind, parallel-group, randomized clinical trial had subjects using the SnF_2 and SHMP or the control dentifrice twice a day for 8 weeks. The SnF_2 and SHMP produced a significant reduction in DH and a mean desensitizing improvement of 71% greater than the sodium fluoride control group.

Risk reduction

Orchardson and Gillam[5] suggest that prevention of DH is not given enough emphasis by dental professionals. Reduction of risk factors should generally be considered when treating any condition. The identification and elimination of such factors should routinely be considered when developing a treatment plan. Risk factors allegedly associated with DH include exposure to erosive substances (eg, acidic beverages) and brushing with an abrasive paste.[44] The effect of chemically erosive substances can be limited by treatment of gastroesophageal reflux disease, limiting consumption of acidic foods and beverages, and avoiding brushing for two to three hours after consumption of acidic substances (or following an episode of gastric reflux). Dietary analysis may be a useful tool in risk assessment.

SUMMARY

Self-applied DH treatments are popular because they are both economical and easy to use. Self-applied products are most commonly found in the form of dentifrices, but

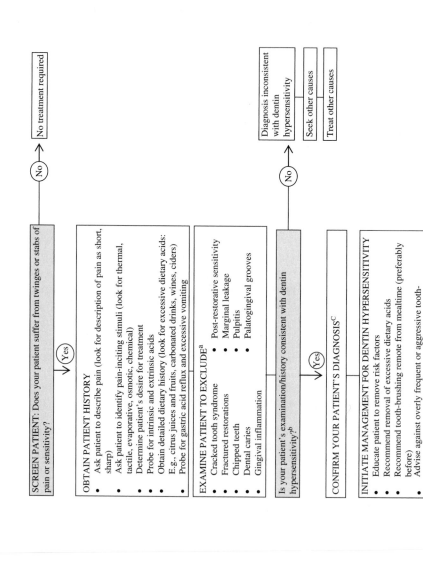

SCREEN PATIENT: Does your patient suffer from twinges or stabs of pain or sensitivity?

No → No treatment required

Yes

OBTAIN PATIENT HISTORY
- Ask patient to describe pain (look for description of pain as short, sharp)
- Ask patient to identify pain-inciting stimuli (look for thermal, tactile, evaporative, osmotic, chemical)
- Determine patient's desire for treatment
- Probe for intrinsic and extrinsic acids
- Obtain detailed dietary history (look for excessive dietary acids: E.g., citrus juices and fruits, carbonated drinks, wines, ciders)
- Probe for gastric acid reflux and excessive vomiting

EXAMINE PATIENT TO EXCLUDE[a]
- Cracked tooth syndrome
- Fractured restorations
- Chipped teeth
- Dental caries
- Gingival inflammation
- Post-restorative sensitivity
- Marginal leakage
- Pulpitis
- Palatogingival grooves

Is your patient's examination/history consistent with dentin hypersensitivity?[b]

No → Diagnosis inconsistent with dentin hypersensitivity

Seek other causes

Treat other causes

Yes

CONFIRM YOUR PATIENT'S DIAGNOSIS[c]

INITIATE MANAGEMENT FOR DENTIN HYPERSENSITIVITY
- Educate patient to remove risk factors
- Recommend removal of excessive dietary acids
- Recommend tooth-brushing remote from mealtime (preferably before)
- Advise against overly frequent or aggressive tooth-brushing/hygiene

Fig. 1. Algorithm for management of DH.

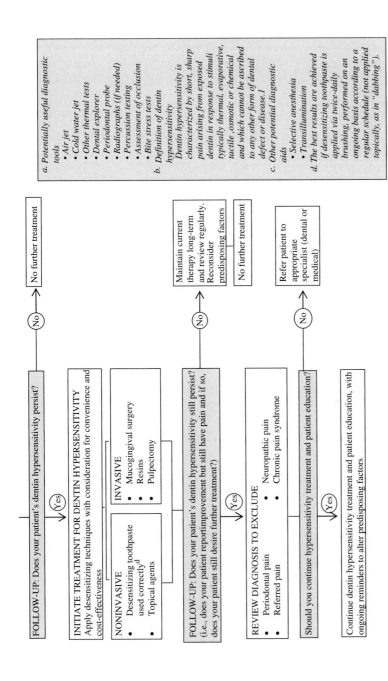

Fig. 1. *(continued)*

gels and solutions are also available over the counter. The disadvantages of self-applied treatments include compliance, difficulty to deliver to specific sites, slow onset of action, and the requirement for continuous use.

Conflicting research findings make it difficult for the practitioner to determine which self-applied product to advise patients to use. There are a number of issues which have plagued research in this area including lack of standardization of stimulus testing and inadequate sample size. The evidence is insufficient to permit the development of evidence-based guidelines for the treatment of DH. Nevertheless, patients will appear in the office tomorrow complaining of DH. Recent guidelines for the management of DH were developed by the Canadian Advisory Board on Dentin Hypersensitivity and are shown in **Fig. 1**.[45] While these also suffer from an underlying deficiency of evidence, they at least offer a logical approach to the patient and are, therefore, recommended for consideration, pending further and better evidence.

REFERENCES

1. Addy M. Etiology and clinical implications of dentine hypersensitivity. Dent Clin North Am 1990;34(3):503–14.
2. Holland GR, Narhi MN, Addy M, et al. Guidelines for the design and conduct of clinical trials on dentine hypersensitivity. J Clin Periodontol 1997;24(11):808–13.
3. Markowitz K, Kim S. The role of selected cations in the desensitization of intradental nerves. Proc Finn Dent Soc 1992;88(Suppl 1):39–54.
4. Hujoel PP. Definitive vs. exploratory periodontal trials: a survey of published studies. J Dent Res 1995;74(8):1453–8.
5. Orchardson R, Gillam DG. Managing dentin hypersensitivity. J Am Dent Assoc 2006;137(7):1028–9 [quiz 990–8].
6. Walters PA. Dentinal hypersensitivity: a review. J Contemp Dent Pract 2005;6(2): 107–17.
7. Jacobsen PL, Bruce G. Clinical dentin hypersensitivity: understanding the causes and prescribing a treatment. J Contemp Dent Pract 2001;2(1):1–12.
8. Bamise CT, Olusile AO, Oginni AO. An analysis of the etiological and predisposing factors related to dentin hypersensitivity. J Contemp Dent Pract 2008;9(5): 52–9.
9. Guyatt G, Jaeschke R, Meade MO, et al. Why study results mislead: bias and random error. In: Guyatt G, Rennie D, Meade MO, et al, editors. Users' guides to the medical literature: a manual for evidence-based clinical practice. New York: McGraw-Hill Medical; 2008. p. 59–66.
10. Guyatt G, Jaeschke R, Prasad K, et al. Summarizing the evidence. In: Guyatt G, Rennie D, Meade MO, et al, editors. Users' guides to the medical literature: a manual for evidence-based clinical practice. New York: McGraw-Hill Medical; 2008. p. 523–54.
11. Markowitz K, Kim S. Hypersensitive teeth. Experimental studies of dentinal desensitizing agents. Dent Clin North Am 1990;34(3):491–501.
12. Gedalia I, Anaise J, Laufer E. Effect of prenatal, preeruptive, and posteruptive strontium administration on dental caries in hamster molars. J Dent Res 1975; 54(6):1240.
13. Spets-Happonen S, Seppa L, Korhonen A, et al. Accumulation of strontium and fluoride in approximal dental plaque and changes in plaque microflora after rinsing with chlorhexidine-fluoride-strontium solution. Oral Dis 1998;4(2):114–9.
14. Foreman JC, Hallett MB, Mongar JL. Movement of strontium ions into mast cells and its relationship to the secretory response. J Physiol 1977;271(1):233–51.

15. Kishore A, Mehrotra KK, Saimbi CS. Effectiveness of desensitizing agents. J Endod 2002;28(1):34–5.
16. Cohen A. Preliminary study of the effects of a strontium chloride dentifrice for the control of hypersensitive teeth. Oral Surg Oral Med Oral Pathol 1961;14:1046–52.
17. Meffert RM, Hoskins SW. Strontium chloride dentifrice to control dental hypersensitivity. Rev Esp Parad 1968;6(2):99–107.
18. Minkoff S, Axelrod S. Efficacy of strontium chloride in dental hypersensitivity. J Periodontol 1987;58(7):470–4.
19. Uchida A, Wakano Y, Fukuyama O, et al. Controlled clinical evaluation of a 10% strontium chloride dentifrice in treatment of dentin hypersensitivity following periodontal surgery. J Periodontol 1980;51(10):578–81.
20. Silverman G, Berman E, Hanna CB, et al. Assessing the efficacy of three dentifrices in the treatment of dentinal hypersensitivity. J Am Dent Assoc 1996;127(2):191–201.
21. Tarbet WJ, Silverman G, Fratarcangelo PA, et al. Home treatment for dentinal hypersensitivity: a comparative study. J Am Dent Assoc 1982;105(2):227–30.
22. Hodosh M. A superior desensitizer—potassium nitrate. J Am Dent Assoc 1974; 88(4):831–2.
23. Kim S. Hypersensitive teeth: desensitization of pulpal sensory nerves. J Endod 1986;12(10):482–5.
24. Greenhill JD, Pashley DH. The effects of desensitizing agents on the hydraulic conductance of human dentin in vitro. J Dent Res 1981;60(3):686–98.
25. Tarbet WJ, Silverman G, Stolman JM, et al. Clinical evaluation of a new treatment for dentinal hypersensitivity. J Periodontol 1980;51(9):535–40.
26. Nagata T, Ishida H, Shinohara H, et al. Clinical evaluation of a potassium nitrate dentifrice for the treatment of dentinal hypersensitivity. J Clin Periodontol 1994; 21(3):217–21.
27. Schiff T, Zhang YP, DeVizio W, et al. A randomized clinical trial of the desensitizing efficacy of three dentifrices. Compend Contin Educ Dent Suppl 2000;(27):4–10 [quiz 28].
28. Sowinski JA, Battista GW, Petrone ME, et al. A new desensitizing dentifrice—an 8-week clinical investigation. Compend Contin Educ Dent Suppl 2000;(27):11–6 [quiz 28].
29. Sowinski JA, Bonta Y, Battista GW, et al. Desensitizing efficacy of colgate sensitive maximum strength and fresh mint sensodyne dentifrices. Am J Dent 2000; 13(3):116–20.
30. Pereira R, Chava VK. Efficacy of a 3% potassium nitrate desensitizing mouthwash in the treatment of dentinal hypersensitivity. J Periodontol 2001;72(12):1720–5.
31. Ayad F, Berta R, De Vizio W, et al. Comparative efficacy of two dentifrices containing 5% potassium nitrate on dentinal sensitivity: a twelve-week clinical study. J Clin Dent 1994;5:97–101.
32. Hu D, Zhang YP, Chaknis P, et al. Comparative investigation of the desensitizing efficacy of a new dentifrice containing 5.5% potassium citrate: an eight-week clinical study. J Clin Dent 2004;15(1):6–10.
33. Chesters R, Kaufman HW, Wolff MS, et al. Use of multiple sensitivity measurements and logit statistical analysis to assess the effectiveness of a potassium citrate–containing dentifrice in reducing dentinal hypersensitivity. J Clin Periodontol 1992;19(4):256–61.
34. Poulsen S, Errboe M, Lescay Mevil Y, et al. Potassium-containing toothpastes for dentine hypersensitivity. Cochrane Database Syst Rev 2006;3:CD001476.
35. Zinner DD, Duany LF, Lutz HJ. A new desensitizing dentifrice: preliminary report. J Am Dent Assoc 1977;95(5):982–5.

36. Collins JF, Perkins L. Clinical evaluation of the effectiveness of three dentifrices in relieving dentin sensitivity. J Periodontol 1984;55(12):720–5.
37. McFall WT Jr, Hamrick SW. Clinical effectiveness of a dentifrice containing fluoride and a citrate buffer system for treatment of dentinal sensitivity. J Periodontol 1987;58(10):701–5.
38. Minkov B, Marmari I, Gedalia I, et al. The effectiveness of sodium fluoride treatment with and without iontophoresis on the reduction of hypersensitive dentin. J Periodontol 1975;46(4):246–9.
39. Tal M, Oron M, Gedalia I, et al. X-ray diffraction and scanning electron microscope investigations of fluoride-treated dentine in man. Arch Oral Biol 1976; 21(5):285–90.
40. Kanouse MC, Ash MM Jr. The effectiveness of a sodium monofluorophosphate dentifrice on dental hypersensitivity. J Periodontol 1969;40(1):38–40.
41. Thrash WJ, Dorman HL, Smith FD. A method to measure pain associated with hypersensitive dentin. J Periodontol 1983;54(3):160–2.
42. Blong MA, Volding B, Thrash WJ, et al. Effects of a gel containing 0.4 percent stannous fluoride on dentinal hypersensitivity. Dent Hyg (Chic) 1985;59(11): 489–92.
43. Schiff T, Saletta L, Baker RA, et al. Desensitizing effect of a stabilized stannous fluoride/sodium hexametaphosphate dentifrice. Compend Contin Educ Dent 2005;26(9 Suppl 1):35–40.
44. Addy M, Hunter ML. Can tooth brushing damage your health? Effects on oral and dental tissues. Int Dent J 2003;53(Suppl 3):177–86.
45. Canadian Advisory Board on Dentin Hypersensitivity. Consensus-based recommendations for the diagnosis and management of dentin hypersensitivity. J Can Dent Assoc 2003;69(4):221–6.

Restoration of Posterior Teeth in Clinical Practice: Evidence Base for Choosing Amalgam Versus Composite

Robert E. Kovarik, DMD, MS

KEYWORDS

- Amalgam • Composite • Posterior restorations • Clinical
- Evidence-based dentistry • Clinical recommendations

CLINICAL PRACTICE IN THE TWENTY-FIRST CENTURY

The restoration of posterior teeth with direct restorations in clinical practice has changed significantly over the past 30 years. Prior to 1980, amalgam was clearly the restoration of choice for use in posterior teeth and was preferred by the vast majority of private practitioners. Both the amalgam alloys and the clinical techniques of placement were longstanding, well-established protocols with an outstanding clinical track record. However, a number of issues began to push clinicians to evaluate alternatives to dental amalgam about 30 years ago. There began a cultural shift in dental consumers that placed a higher value on esthetics and natural-appearing restorations. This increased demand for esthetic restorations has grown over 30 years and is strong today. Another change was the increased consideration of the potential health issues associated with mercury in amalgam. Although there has never been a scientific study that directly links the clinical use of amalgam to any health concern, nevertheless it has been shown that mercury does indeed leach out of amalgam restorations and adds to the biologic burden of mercury on the human system, along with mercury doses that are derived from food and air. Finally, increasing concerns about the environmental impact of mercury waste from dental offices have driven some dentists away from the clinical use of amalgam as well.

More dentists began to utilize resin composite for posterior restorations in the 1970s; however, there were clinical issues that limited its use, including wear, color

Department of Oral Health Science, University of Kentucky College of Dentistry, Room 402, Health Science Research Building, 800 Rose Street, Lexington, KY 40536-0297, USA
E-mail address: rekova2@uky.edu

Dent Clin N Am 53 (2009) 71–76
doi:10.1016/j.cden.2008.11.001
0011-8532/08/$ – see front matter

dental.theclinics.com

stability, leakage, recurrent caries, and difficulty in placement technique.[1–6] Even in the 1980s, 89% of practitioners in the United States reported using amalgam as the restoration of choice in their clinical practice.[7] The use of resin composite has changed dramatically since the report by Pink and colleagues.[7] In the past decade, there has been a large shift toward using resin composite for posterior restorations. Today, it is more commonly placed than amalgam restorations. The shift in clinical practice occurred for a number of reasons. First, there is a perception that patients prefer esthetics restorations and that belief is supported by the literature. One study found that a majority of patients prefer a tooth-colored material (composite), even when informed that the clinical longevity will be shorter than that of amalgam.[8] In the same study, dentists more frequently wanted to place the material with better clinical performance. Dentists were more influenced by longevity while patients were more influenced by esthetics. Second, dentists themselves have the perception that materials and bonding systems have significantly improved. Third, continued environmental and health concerns about mercury in dental amalgam have pushed many patients and some practitioners to try and use less amalgam.[9–12] In some countries there are regulatory controls that limit or eliminate the use of amalgam. Finally, dentists have improved methods of composite placement, which improve contour and proximal contacts. These placement methods (eg, the use of sectional, contoured matrices with bitine rings) are now taught by most dental schools and easily implemented by practitioners. The shift from amalgam dominance in practice to composite has been remarkable.

EVIDENCE BASE FOR MATERIAL OF CHOICE FOR DIRECT POSTERIOR RESTORATIONS

Practitioners have perceived clinical improvements in posterior resin composite restorations and have significantly increased the use of resin composite for posterior applications. But is there a real evidence base for this drastic swing in the use of resin composites in posterior restorations? The use of evidence-based clinical decision making in dentistry is still in its infancy. Most dental practitioners do not rely on high levels of evidence, but rather base clinical decisions on opinion and individual case observations.[13] The gold standard for evidence-base in clinical practice is the randomized, controlled clinical trial or a systematic review based on a number of such trials.

There have been several thorough reviews in the literature comparing the use of amalgam and composite use in direct posterior restorations.[14–22] A large number of these studies would indicate that resin composite used clinically as a posterior restoration performed equal to or better than amalgam. One thorough recent review of the literature summarized that the yearly failure rate of composite was 0% to 9%, while the yearly failure rate of amalgam was 0% to 7%.[7] Other studies actually show lower failure rates for resin composite than amalgam.[23] However, using an evidence-based approach, one must look at the literature very carefully. A comprehensive electronic and hard copy search was made, using PubMed, the Cochrane Library, and similar resources.

SEARCH RESULTS

Virtually all studies that were located on posterior resin composites and amalgam were either retrospective case series, retrospective epidemiologic studies, or prospective, nonrandomized studies. Retrospective studies on longevity have rated the clinical performance of posterior resin composites very close to amalgam restorations.[23–26] One prospective trial also found no difference in longevity of amalgam or composite but was based on only 38 subjects.[27] These types of studies are very susceptible to various forms of bias and confounding variables that are impossible to account for. For example, a prospective, nonrandomized study that allows the patient to choose his or her restoration of choice (composite versus amalgam) may be open to a bias as a result of oral hygiene. The group that chooses the esthetic tooth colored restoration may also be a group that generally has higher oral care expectations and lower plaque scores. Such a systematic difference between the test and control subjects may influence the outcome of the study. Such confounding factors, both known and unknown, are presumably compensated for by randomly allocating a sufficiently large number of subjects to test and control sides. Another way to compensate for inter-subject differences is to employ a split-mouth design, in which clinically similar lesions on contralateral teeth are randomly allocated to receive either amalgam or composite. The comparison is thus between the restorations within the mouth of the same patient.

Another study design issue that has recently been questioned is the validity of "university-based" research verses "practice-based" research. The vast majority (virtually all) studies of longevity of composite versus amalgam—particularly prospective studies—have been done in university settings. Restoration locations in these studies follow a strict placement protocol under rubber dam isolation, with no time constraints in placement, and by the most meticulous operators who teach operative dentistry and are detail oriented. Often, the study populations are university faculty, staff, and students with high educational levels and high oral health IQs. An argument being made is that these placement conditions and study subjects are not realistic to what is seen in private practice. As such, new studies of materials, techniques, and longevity are being planned in "practice-based" networks, thereby yielding data that is truly a result of clinical practice in a private practice setting.[28–32]

In evaluating the evidence-base for posterior composites or amalgam, the vast majority of the literature on the use of amalgam or composite in posterior teeth is very low-level evidence (see the articles "Evidence-based curriculum reform: the Kentucky experience" and "Evidence-based dentistry and the concept of harm" by Thomas and colleagues elsewhere in this issue, which describe the hierarchy of evidence). There are numerous bench-top studies and expert opinion that have evaluated wear, microleakage, marginal integrity, and shrinkage; and while these studies show plausible reasons that these materials will perform well, these studies would not dictate use in private practice. As noted elsewhere in this issue (see the article "Evidence-based dentistry and the concept of harm" by Thomas and colleagues), such information constitutes a very low level of evidence. Likewise, there are many retrospective case reports and case series in the literature evaluating reasons for failure and estimating yearly failure rates; these studies are prone to bias and results of these studies are often conflicting. There are far fewer prospective, controlled studies in the literature on amalgam or composite restorations (level 3 and 4). What is needed to make such clinical decisions are randomized, controlled trials (RCTs) or, preferably, systematic reviews based on multiple RCTs.

A search was undertaken to find trials that might provide a stronger evidentiary basis on which to make a decision between the two materials. PubMed was searched using the keywords composite, amalgam, clinical, and longevity. In this search, results were limited to clinical trials. Two RCTs were identified that directly compared amalgams and composites for posterior restorations. Unfortunately, the study populations in both were children, which ultimately limits the generalizability with regard to an adult population. However, these studies provide the strongest evidence on which to base clinical decisions.

The first of these RCTs is from the New England Children's Amalgam Trial. The primary outcome that was examined in this study was the safety of mercury-containing amalgam restorations in children.[33] A secondary outcome that was examined was longevity of posterior restorations after 2 to 5 years of follow-up. A total of 534 children (average age 7.9 years old) were randomly assigned to receive posterior amalgam or posterior composites and a total of 1,262 restorations were placed. Replacement of restorations were more frequently needed for the resin composites (14.9%) than for amalgam restoration (10.8%); however, this difference was not statistically significant in the random effects survival mode ($P = 0.45$). This study also noted that while replacement rates were similar (14.9% versus 10.8%), the reasons for replacement were quite different. Composites demonstrated more recurrent caries and required repair more often.

The second RCT was also part of a large RCT with the primary outcome measure being the safety of mercury-containing restoratives.[34] This study randomly assigned 472 children (ages 8–12) to receive either amalgam or composite restorations in their posterior teeth. A total of 1,748 restorations were followed for 7 years. Overall, 10.1% of all restorations failed over the 7-year trial (5.6% of amalgams and 14.5% of composites). The 7-year survival rate for amalgams was 94.4%, while the survival rate of composites was 85.5%. This RCT agreed with the other available RCT that recurrent caries was much more common in composites than in amalgams (composite recurrent caries were +12.7%, while amalgam recurrent caries were 3.7%). The relative risk of recurrent caries was 3.5 (95% confidence interval of 2.3–5.1, $P<0.0001$).

These two randomized, controlled clinical studies demonstrate clearly that amalgam has higher survival than composite for posterior restorations, and there is much more secondary decay associated with resin composite than amalgam in posterior restorations. These two findings should be conveyed to patients who are receiving restorations in their posterior teeth, so that patients can make decisions with their provider that are informed decisions.

As noted previously, these two studies are the strongest evidence now available on this topic. However, the study populations were elementary school children and the results may not be entirely applicable to adults. Trials are needed to assess the longevity of composite and amalgam restorations in a large sample of adult patients. As an aside, it may be worthwhile to evaluate the safety of composite vis-à-vis amalgam restorations. While there have long been concerns about the safety of amalgam because of its mercury content, recently, concerns have been voiced concerning potential health effects of bisphenol A, a component of some composite resins. Future trials will be needed to clarify these issues.

SUMMARY

There is no doubt that the use of resin composite in posterior restorations has become common in dental practices in the United States and the world today. While there are abundant retrospective and prospective case series showing similar longevity of amalgam and composite in posterior restorations, the higher level of evidence (RCTs) indicates that indeed, amalgam is superior in its clinical performance. Not only is the expected longevity two to three times longer, but failure of posterior composites is much more likely to be associated with recurrent caries, a fact that may influence the long-term survival of the tooth itself. This real endpoint, tooth loss, has never been studied with respect to placement of amalgam versus resin composite in the posterior dentition, but would ultimately have more clinical relevance than simply looking at replacement rates.

REFERENCES

1. Phillips RW, Avery DR, Mehra R, et al. Observations on a composite resin for class II restorations: two-year report. J Prosthet Dent 1972;28(2):164–9.

2. Osborne JW, Gale EN, Ferguson GW. One-year and two-year clinical evaluation of a composite resin vs. amalgam. J Prosthet Dent 1973;30(5):795–800.
3. Phillips RW, Avery DR, Mehra R, et al. Observations on a composite resin for class II restorations: three-year report. J Prosthet Dent 1973;30(6):891–7.
4. Williams DF. Dental materials: 1973 literature review. J Dent 1975;3(2):51–67.
5. Elderton RJ. The prevalence of failure of restorations: a literature review. J Dent 1976;4(5):207–10.
6. Waters NE. Dental materials: 1974 literature review. Part I. J Dent 1976;4(2): 51–67.
7. Pink FE, Minden NJ, Simmonds S. Decisions of practitioners regarding placement of amalgam and composite restorations in general practice settings. Oper Dent 1994;19(4):127–32.
8. Espelid I, Cairns J, Askildsen JE, et al. Preferences over dental restorative materials among young patients and dental professionals. Eur J Oral Sci 2006;114(1): 15–21.
9. Hiltz M. The environmental impact of dentistry. J Can Dent Assoc 2007;73(1): 59–62.
10. Jokstad A, Fan PL. Amalgam waste management. Int Dent J 2006;56(3):147–53.
11. Burk JW. The impact of mercury on the environment. J Calif Dent Assoc 2004; 32(11):885 [discussion: 885].
12. Mohapatra SP, Nikolova I, Mitchell A. Managing mercury in the great lakes: an analytical review of abatement policies. J Environ Manage 2007;83(1):80–92.
13. Haj-Ali RN, et al. Utilization of evidence-based informational resources for clinical decisions related to posterior composite restorations. J Dent Educ 2005;69(11): 1251–6.
14. Le Roux AR, Lachman N. Dental composite materials: highlighting the problem of wear for posterior restorations. SADJ 2007;62(8):342–4.
15. Mitchell RJ, Koike M, Okabe T. Posterior amalgam restorations—usage, regulation, and longevity. Dent Clin North Am 2007;51(3):573–89, v.
16. Giachetti L, et al. A review of polymerization shrinkage stress: current techniques for posterior direct resin restorations. J Contemp Dent Pract 2006;7(4): 79–88.
17. Stein PS, et al. Composite resin in medicine and dentistry. J Long Term Eff Med Implants 2005;15(6):641–54.
18. Wahl MJ. A resin alternative for posterior teeth: questions and answers on dental amalgam. Dent Update 2003;30(5):256–62.
19. Burgess JO, Walker T, Davidson JM. Posterior resin-based composite: review of the literature. Pediatr Dent 2002;24(5):465–79.
20. Hondrum SO. The longevity of resin-based composite restorations in posterior teeth. Gen Dent 2000;48(4):398–404.
21. Wilson NH, Dunne SM, Gainsford ID. Current materials and techniques for direct restorations in posterior teeth. Part 2: Resin composite systems. Int Dent J 1997; 47(4):185–93.
22. Leinfelder KF. Posterior composite resins: the materials and their clinical performance. J Am Dent Assoc 1995;126(5):663–4, 667–8, 671–2 passim.
23. Opdam NJ, Bronkhorst EM, Roeters JM, et al. A retrospective clinical study on longevity of posterior composite and amalgam restorations. Dent Mater 2007; 23(1):2–8.
24. Manhart J, Chen H, Hamm G, et al. Buonocore memorial lecture. Review of the clinical survival of direct and indirect restorations in posterior teeth of the permanent dentition. Oper Dent 2004;29(5):481–508.

25. Hickel R, Manhart J. Longevity of restorations in posterior teeth and reasons for failure. J Adhes Dent 2001;3(1):45–64.
26. Mjor IA, Dahl JE, Moorhead JE. Age of restorations at replacement in permanent teeth in general dental practice. Acta Odontol Scand 2000;58(3):97–101.
27. da Rosa Rodolpho PA, Cenci MS, Donassollo TA, et al. A clinical evaluation of posterior composite restorations: 17-year findings. J Dent 2006;34(7):427–35.
28. Chattopadhyay A, Arevalo O, Sohn W. Understanding measurement of dental diseases and research participation in practice set-up. Dent Clin North Am 2008;52(2):367–86, vii.
29. Gilbert GH, Williams OD, Rindal DB, et al. The creation and development of the dental practice-based research network. J Am Dent Assoc 2008;139(1):74–81.
30. Bayne SC. Dental restorations for oral rehabilitation—testing of laboratory properties versus clinical performance for clinical decision making. J Oral Rehabil 2007; 34(12):921–32.
31. Mjor IA. Practice-based dental research. J Oral Rehabil 2007;34(12):913–20.
32. Veitz-Keenan A, Berkowitz GS, Brandes I, et al. Practice-based research networks. N Y State Dent J 2007;73(3):14–5.
33. Bellinger DC, Trachtenberg F, Barregard L, et al. Neuropsychological and renal effects of dental amalgam in children: a randomized clinical trial. JAMA 2006; 295(15):1775–83.
34. DeRouen TA, Martin MD, Leroux BG, et al. Neurobehavioral effects of dental amalgam in children: a randomized clinical trial. JAMA 2006;295(15):1784–92.

Evidenced-Based Decision Making: The Third Molar

Richard H. Haug, DDS[a],*, Jihaad Abdul-Majid, BS[a],
George H. Blakey, DDS[b], Raymond P. White, DDS[b]

KEYWORDS

- Parameters of care - Third molars - Alveolar osteitis
- Anesthesia - Parasthesia - Infection

Oral and maxillofacial surgery is a surgical specialty based in dentistry and founded upon science. Scientific research is the foundation upon which oral and maxillofacial surgeons are trained, and decisions are made. This has included education and decision-making in the lecture hall, in the operating room, while on rounds, and in the clinical setting. This science, research, and publication are the evidence with which education and decisions are based. While traditional teaching and decision making has included a review and interpretation of the literature, the American Association of Oral and Maxillofacial Surgeons (AAOMS) has been at the forefront of formal evidence-based dentistry with such projects as the *Parameters of Care: Clinical Practice Guidelines for Oral and Maxillofacial Surgeons*, now in its fourth edition;[1–4] the AAOMS Outcomes Assessment Program;[5,6] the AAOMS Third Molar Clinical Trial;[7–37] and the AAOMS "White Paper on Third Molar Data," which is based upon a review of the current literature.[38] This article reviews these evidence-based resources to provide a consensus of opinion for the management of the third molar.

THE AMERICAN ASSOCIATION OF ORAL AND MAXILLOFACIAL SURGEONS PARAMETERS OF CARE

Recognizing the need to identify and support evidenced-based decision making, the AAOMS in 1986 created a 22-member committee to develop criteria and standards of care for oral and maxillofacial surgery. The product of its first labors was the original *Parameters of Care.*[1] This document contained a section on dentoalveolar surgery that addressed the management of third molars. The publication is now in its fourth

[a] University of Kentucky College of Dentistry, D-136, 800 Rose Street, Room, Lexington, KY 40536-0297, USA
[b] Department of Oral and Maxillofacial Surgery, School of Dentistry, University of North Carolina at Chapel Hill, Chapel Hill, NC 27599-7450, USA
* Corresponding author.
E-mail address: rhhaug2@uky.edu (R.H. Haug).

Dent Clin N Am 53 (2009) 77–96
doi:10.1016/j.cden.2008.09.004
0011-8532/08/$ – see front matter © 2009 Elsevier Inc. All rights reserved.

dental.theclinics.com

edition, after sustained scrutiny by thousands of oral and maxillofacial surgeons, other specialty organizations, and communities of interest, and is endorsed by 44 international oral and maxillofacial surgical societies. The current section that addresses third molars is based upon a review of more than 100 peer-reviewed publications. It contains, in outline form, indications for therapy, therapeutic goals, factors affecting risk, therapeutic standards, and outcome assessment indices. They are reproduced as **Boxes 1–5**. This outline addresses the management of third molars from the time the patient enters the office, through diagnosis and definitive therapy, to completion of the case.

THE AMERICAN ASSOCIATION OF ORAL AND MAXILLOFACIAL SURGEONS AGE-RELATED THIRD-MOLAR STUDY

In response to the ever-changing health care marketplace and increased presence of managed care, the AAOMS, in 1995, commissioned a special subcommittee for outcomes assessment. The charge of this group was to identify high-volume and high-profile oral and maxillofacial surgical procedures, and then to objectively assess their management and the outcomes of each therapeutic modality. One of the first projects was to review the demographics and postoperative results after the removal of third molars in an older population.[5] This was meant to be the largest prospective evaluation of patients 25 years of age or older who had third molars removed. During this study,

---

Box 1
Indications for therapy for third molars

Pain

Pericoronitis

Nonrestorable carious tooth

Facilitation of the management of, or limitation of progression of, periodontal disease

Nontreatable pulpal or periapical lesion

Acute or chronic infection

Ectopic position

Abnormalities of tooth size or shape precluding normal function

Facilitation of prosthetic rehabilitation

Facilitation of orthodontic tooth movement and promotion of dental stability

Tooth in the line of fracture

Tooth involved in tumor resection

Pathology associated with tooth follicle

Tooth interfering with orthognathic or reconstructive jaw surgery

Preventive or prophylactic removal, when indicated, for patients with medical or surgical conditions or treatments

Clinical findings of pulp exposure by dental caries

Clinical findings of fractured tooth or teeth

Internal or external resorption of tooth or adjacent teeth

Impacted tooth

Need for donor transplant

> **Box 2**
> **Possible therapeutic goals of third-molar removal**
>
> To prevent pathology
>
> To preserve periodontal health of adjacent teeth
>
> To optimize prosthetic rehabilitation
>
> To optimize management or healing of jaw fracture
>
> To optimize orthodontic results
>
> To aid in tumor resection
>
> To provide healthy oral and maxillofacial environment for patients undergoing radiation therapy, chemotherapy, organ transplantation, or placement of alloplastic implants or other devices
>
> To prevent complications of orthognathic surgery

3760 patients had 8333 third molars removed by 63 surgeons. Age, gender, American Society of Anesthesiologists (ASA) status, chronic conditions, medical risk factors, and the preoperative description of the third molars were recorded. Intraoperative and post-operative complications were also recorded and frequencies tabulated. From among the 3760 patients (52.0% male; 48.0% female), all were 25 years of age or older, with 9845 third molars of which 8333 were removed. A majority of the patients involved in the study were healthy (72.5%). Hypertension and chronic heart disease were the most frequently encountered chronic conditions, representing approximately 10.2% and 4.8% of the patient population, respectively. At least one risk factor, including smoking (16.3%), medications (9.3%) and alcohol use (9.0%), was encountered in

> **Box 3**
> **Specific factors affecting risk for third-molar removal**
>
> Size and density of supporting bone
>
> Anatomic relationships of tooth or teeth to:
>
>   Maxillary antrum and nasal cavity
>
>   Adjacent nerves
>
>   Adjacent teeth
>
>   Other significant anatomic structures
>
> Anatomic tooth position
>
> Tooth root anatomy
>
> Status of adjacent teeth
>
> Ankylosis of tooth or teeth
>
> Presence of associate jaw fracture
>
> Accessibility
>
> Limited access to oral cavity
>
> Systemic drugs, such as bisphosphonates
>
> Radiation therapy to surgical sites

Box 4
Indicated therapeutic standards for third-molar removal

History

Clinical examination

Imaging examination

Surgical removal

Surgical exposure

Surgical repositioning, reimplantation, or transplantation

Surgical periodontics

Endodontic therapy

Coronectomy

Marsupialization of associated soft tissue pathology with observation

Observation in cases of unerupted teeth completely covered by bone

Instructions for posttreatment care

---

greater than 29.2% of the patients. Almost one quarter (20.5%–27.0%) of third molars were absent upon initial patient evaluation. Caries (17.6%–20.3%), periodontal disease (11.6%–17.6%), and infection (6.3%–16.7%) were the most frequently encountered preoperative diagnoses. Intraoperative complications occurred with a frequency of less than 1%. There were no deaths or compromised airways. No patient suffered a mandibular fracture and only 1 a maxillary alveolar fracture. Alveolar osteitis was the most commonly encountered postoperative problem and occurred with a frequency of about 2 or 3 in 1000 encounters for maxillary third molars (0.2%–0.3%) and slightly

---

Box 5
Known risks and complications for third-molar removal

Acute or chronic infection

Alveolar osteitis

Acute or chronic osteomyelitis

Injury to adjacent teeth or soft tissues

Presence of foreign body in surgical site

Osteonecrosis, osteoradionecrosis

Presence of portion of tooth intentionally left in alveolus

Presence of portion of tooth unintentionally left in alveolus

Presence of bone fragment or sequestra in surgical site

Exposure of alveolar bone

Mandibular or maxillary fracture

Condition that requires unplanned additional surgery

Oroantral or nasal fistula formation

Displacement of tooth, tooth fragments, or foreign bodies into adjacent anatomic sites

Persistent or new pathology

---

more than 1 in 10 (11.9%–12.7%) for mandibular third molars. Acute or chronic infections occurred with a frequency of 0.0% to 1.0 % per patient. Inferior alveolar nerve anesthesia/paresthesia was encountered postoperatively with a frequency of 1.1% to 1.7%. Lingual nerve anesthesia/paresthesia occurred with a lower frequency (0.3%), between three and six times that for inferior alveolar anesthesia/paresthesia. Lastly, for almost a third of patients (31.2%–34.1%), inconvenience associated with the extraction was minimal. These patients neither missed work nor had normal activities curtailed. The study concluded that third-molar surgery in patients 25 years old or older is associated with minimal morbidity, a low incidence of postoperative complication, and a minimal impact on the patient's quality of life.

The next paper in the series was designed to estimate the frequency of complications after third-molar surgery, with age as the primary risk factor.[6] This was a prospective cohort study of a sample of subjects having at least one third-molar extracted. The predictor variables were categorized as demographic, health status, anatomic, and pathologic. The outcome variable was overall complications, including both intraoperative and postoperative complications. Appropriate univariate and bivariate statistics were computed. A multiple logistic regression model was used to evaluate the simultaneous effects of multiple covariates. The overall complication rate was 19%. Age above 25 years, gender, ASA classification, number of preoperatively identified risk factors for complication, impaction level of the third molar, evidence of periodontal disease, preoperative infection, and evidence of any pathology associated with the third molar were associated with complications ($P \leq .15$).

THE AMERICAN ASSOCIATION OF ORAL AND MAXILLOFACIAL SURGEONS THIRD-MOLAR CLINICAL TRIAL

In the late 1980s and early 1990s, the AAOMS invested approximately $2 million in its own dues to conduct research regarding the consequences of the removal of third molars versus their intended permanent retention. From the standpoint of scientific validity, one could question the bias of self-funded research. It is up to the reader to conclude for himself or herself the scientific integrity of the researchers and the investigation. The result has been more than 30 peer-reviewed publications that are summarized in the paragraphs to follow. The rationale for the study was that over 95% of 18-year-olds in the United States have third molars and many are nonfunctional. It is estimated at least 60% will develop pathology, usually caries, periodontitis, or pericoronitis. Thus the study was designed to obtain data to assist patients in decisions regarding third-molar treatment by researching the incidence of third-molar pathology in patients who enrolled with no symptoms. Inclusion criteria included four asymptomatic third molars with adjacent second molars, age 14 to 45 years, ASA categories I and II, American Academy of Periodontology (AAP) categories 1 through 3, and a willingness to commit to study design. Exclusion criteria included ASA III or IV, AAP 4, a history of treatment of a psychiatric disorder within 12 months, or pregnancy. Data were collected from enrolled patients at annual visits until data extending over at least 5 years were collected from each patient, with an attempt to reach 10-year results. The details of the annual and interim clinical visits are listed as **Boxes 6 and 7**.

Recovery After Third Molar Surgery

Numerous studies have been conducted to evaluate patients' perceptions of recovery after third-molar surgery. In one study, 201 patients between ages 13 and 37 underwent surgical removal of third molars.[7] Each patient was given a 21-item Health

---

Box 6
Annual periodontal clinical analysis

Full-mouth probe

Bleeding

Plaque index

Gingival crevicular fluid sampled for inflammatory mediators prostaglandin E2 and IL-β

Subgingival plaque sampled for DNA analysis of microorganisms

Vertical bitewings taken for alveolar bone and tooth position

Panoramic radiograph taken for tooth position and pathology

Surgeon assessment

Patient perception

Dental prophylaxis after data collection

Related Quality Of Life (HRQOL) instrument to be completed each postoperative day for 14 days. The instrument was designed to assess patients' perception of pain, oral function, general activity measures, and other symptoms. The impact of each predictor variable, such as age, gender, and length of surgery on recovery, was assessed. On postoperative day (POD) 1, 63.5% of patients reported their worst pain as severe at some time during the day. On POD 7, only 15% of patients reported their worst pain as severe. Twenty-nine percent reported average pain as severe on POD 1, decreasing to 5.5% by POD 7. Patients assumed a normal lifestyle on POD 5. A surgery time of 30 or more minutes, having all third molars below the occlusal plane, and being female were factors related to prolonged recovery period.

Another study surveyed 630 healthy patients to evaluate average HRQOL and clinical recovery after third-molar surgery.[8] Patients had a median age of 21 and median operating time of 30 minutes. The survey was completed on each postsurgery day for 14 days. The instrument assessed perception of recovery in pain, lifestyle, oral function, and other symptoms related to the procedure. Twenty-two percent of

---

Box 7
Interim periodontal clinical analysis if symptomatic

Full-mouth probed

Bleeding noted

Plaque index measured

Gingival crevicular fluid sampled for inflammatory mediators prostaglandin E2 and IL- β

Subgingival plaque sampled for DNA analysis of microorganisms

Vertical bitewings taken for alveolar bone and tooth position

Panoramic radiograph taken for tooth position and pathology

Additional treatment specific to presenting condition documented

Patient encouraged to continue in trial even if third molars removed

the patients were treated for delayed healing after surgery. Recovery from pain was delayed relative to other HRQOL measures.

Risk factors associated with prolonged recovery and delayed healing after third-molar surgery were evaluated with HRQOL and clinical outcome data after removal of all four third molars.[9] This analysis included 547 subjects who were between 14 and 40 years of age. Patients completed two pages of HRQOL diary each postsurgery day for 14 days. The criteria selected for outcomes that separated patients with prolonged recovery from those without. Delayed clinical healing was indicated when the patient had at least one postsurgery visit with treatment. Patients who were female, older than 18 years, and presenting with both lower third molars below the occlusal plane had greater odds of delayed HRQOL recovery. The odds of delayed clinical recovery were higher for patients who were female, who had previous third-molar symptoms, or whose surgery was difficult, according to the surgeon's evaluation.

The impact of intravenous antibiotics on recovery after third-molar surgery was evaluated in a study that included 56 patients of at least 18 years of age with all four third molars below the occlusal plane.[10] Each patient was given intravenous antibiotics just before third-molar surgery. Clinical and HRQOL outcomes of 56 patients were compared with a nonconcurrent control group of 60 patients who did not receive antibiotics. The control group was selected using the same surgical protocol as that for the antibiotic group. The incidence of delayed clinical recovery was defined as a postsurgery visit with treatment. The incidence of delayed clinical recovery was higher in the control group than in the antibiotic group. In the antibiotic group, 4% had one postsurgery visit with treatment and none had two visits. In the control group without antibiotics, 28% had at least one postsurgery visit with treatment and 13% had at least two postsurgery visits with treatment. No statistically significant differences in HRQOL outcomes were found between the two groups. Intravenous antibiotics at surgery improved clinical recovery, but not HRQOL recovery, for targeted higher-risk patients.

The impact of intravenous corticosteroids on patients with a high risk for delayed recovery was evaluated in a study comparing two groups of 60 adult patients each, each patient with four third molars below the occlusal plane.[11] Patients in group 1 were given intravenous corticosteroids immediately before surgery: 37 were given 8 mg of dexamethasone sodium phosphate; 23 were given 40 mg of methylprednisolone sodium succinate. Patients in group 2 were not given steroids. Patients were each given a diary to record their perceptions of recovery in four categories: pain, lifestyle, oral function, and other symptoms. Recovery was defined as the number of days before patient feels little or no trouble or pain. Delayed recovery was defined as a postsurgery visit with treatment. The incidence of delayed clinical recovery (postsurgery visit with treatment) was higher in the control group than the corticosteroid group. In the corticosteroid group, 10% had one postsurgery visit with treatment. In the control group, 28% had one postsurgery visit with treatment. Compared with the control group, patients in the corticosteroid group were bothered less on postoperative day 1 and sleep was improved on postoperative days 1 through 4. Corticosteroids reduced time of recovery by at least 1 day for pain, lifestyle, and oral function.

The impact of delayed healing was evaluated using recovery data for 547 healthy patients between the ages of 14 and 40 after the removal of four third molars.[12] Data was obtained from patients with the HRQOL instrument, which included domains for lifestyle, oral function, and pain items. The data assessed recovery for each of 14 days postsurgery. Prevalence ratios (PR) with 95% confidence intervals were calculated to compare the prevalence of delayed HRQOL recovery between participants with delayed clinical healing and those without. For patients with delayed clinical healing, the prevalence of delayed recovery for lifestyle nearly doubled (PR 1.7). A higher proportion of those with delayed clinical healing also reported delayed oral function recovery (PR 1.8), late symptoms recovery (PR 2.0), and delayed resolution of pain (PR 1.6). Significant average differences were found between those with delayed clinical healing and those without for sensory intensity of pain and unpleasantness of pain from postsurgery day 3 through day 14.

The impact of topical minocycline on recovery after third-molar surgery was evaluated by examining 63 patients at least 18 years of age, with all four third molars below the occlusal plane.[13] These patients were treated with topical minocycline during third-molar surgery and topical minocycline was placed sequentially in bony defects after third-molar removal. The 63 patients were compared with a control group of 60 patients who did not receive antibiotics. The control group was selected using the same protocol as that for the antibiotic group. Delayed clinical recovery was defined as a postsurgery visit with treatment. The incidence of delayed clinical recovery was significantly lower in the minocycline group compared with that for the control group. In the minocycline group, 10% had one postsurgery visit with treatment and none had two visits. In the control group, 28% had at least one postsurgery visit with treatment and 13% had at least two postsurgery visits with treatment. Recovery time to "no" or "little trouble" with chewing and mouth opening significantly improved in the minocycline group.

To determine if the proximity of a lower third molar to the inferior alveolar canal is a predictor of delayed recovery, data was taken for 579 patients who underwent removal of lower third molars. Radiographic findings were used to identify patients with at least one mandibular third molar below the occlusal plane.[14] Outcomes for patients with one or more radiographic sign indicating the proximity of a lower third molar to the inferior alveolar canal were compared with those with none. After surgery, a questionnaire designed to assess HRQOL recovery was given to each patient to complete daily for 14 days. No significant differences were found between the groups for delayed clinical recovery. However, odds significantly increased for delayed HRQOL recovery for worst pain, lifestyle, and oral function for those patients with close proximity of a third molar to the inferior alveolar canal.

To further develop an understanding of recovery after third-molar surgery, clinical and quality-of-life data pre- and postsurgery were taken from 63 patients with all four third molars below the occlusal plane.[15] During third-molar surgery, each patient was treated with topical minocycline to reduce the incidence of delayed clinical healing. Each patient was given a global Oral Health Impact Profile 14 (OHIP-14) and an HRQOL instrument to assess their recovery. Prevalence, extent, and severity of OHIP-14 scores were calculated pre- and postsurgery for days 1, 7, and 14. The percentage of patients who reported clinically relevant responses detrimental to their quality of life from HRQOL was reported for the same time frame. The median surgery time was 27 minutes with 72% of patients requiring bone removal from both lower third molars. Surgeons gave surgeries an average rating of 14 for difficulty on a scale in which the most difficult surgery is rated 28. Delayed clinical healing was found in 10% of patients. OHIP-14 items "fairly often" or "very often" increased from presurgery to postsurgery day 1, and then decreased on postsurgery day 7 and postsurgery day 14. Clinical (delayed healing) and Oral Health-Related Quality of Life addressed distinctly different outcomes, adding information that could not be assessed by one instrument alone.

Data was taken from 358 patients treated between 1997 and 2002 to determine if completeness of the root formation of lower third molars affected recovery after third-molar surgery. Thus, the root development of each mandibular third molar was assessed.[16] Patients were categorized as those with complete root formation (both mandibular third molars had 100% complete roots) or as those with incomplete root formation (at least one mandibular third molar not completely formed). Patients were evaluated on whether or not they experienced a delay in recovery. Removing third molars when lower third-molar roots were incomplete conferred no advantage or disadvantage in recovery compared with surgery with roots complete.

Epidemiologic/Population Studies

Several epidemiologic/population studies are cited to evaluate the relationship between third molars and periodontal pathology. In the first of these studies cited in this article, data were obtained on 5831 patients between the ages of 18 and 34 from the Third National Health and Nutrition Examination Survey. The presence of a visible third molar was determined.[17] The presence of periodontal disease was assessed in two randomly selected quadrants (one maxillary, one mandibular) by gingival index, pocket depth, and attachment level on mesiobuccal and buccal sites on up to seven teeth per quadrant (excluding third molars). Associations were determined using odd ratios and 95% confidence intervals. Visible third molar was associated with twice the odds of pocket depth of 5 mm or more on adjacent second molar with controls for other factors. Smoking, age between 25 and 34 years, and African American race were also associated with pocket depth of 5 mm or more.

In a study evaluating older Americans, data were obtained from the Atherosclerosis Risk in Communities Study between 1996 and 1999.[18] Data included 6793 persons between 52 and 74 years of age. The independent variable was visual presence or absence of a third molar. The dependent variable was an assessment of periodontal disease as measured by pocket depth of 5 mm or more. Periodontal measures included gingival recession, pocket depth, and attachment level on six sites per tooth on all other teeth. Second molars were compared for periodontal pathology based on the presence or absence of a visible third molar in same quadrant. Visible third molar was associated with 1.5 times the odds of pocket depth of 5 mm or more on the adjacent second molar with controls for other factors. Male gender, older age, smoking, and irregular/episodic dental visits were associated with pocket depth of 5 mm or more.

Data were taken from a subsample of patients with dental exams in the Piedmont 65+ study to assess third-molar periodontal pathology and caries experience in older adults.[19] All visible teeth were examined and periodontal probing (pocket depth) measures were taken at mesiobuccal and buccal/facial sites. Data on caries experience were taken by visual-tactile examination. This subsample of 342 subjects had a mean age of 73 with at least one visible third molar that could be examined. Pocket depth measures were available for 276 of these subjects. Sixty-three percent of the 342 subjects with at least one visible third molar were African American and 57% were female. Forty-nine percent of 197 subjects with caries experience had affected third molars compared with 87% in non–third molars. Third-molar caries experience was associated with non–third-molar experience. Clinical attachment level greater then 3 mm at enrollment in third molars was found in 68% of subjects and in 96% of subjects for non–third molars. With one exception, clinical attachment level 3 mm or more in third molars was associated with clinical attachment level 3 mm or more elsewhere in the mouth. Seventeen percent of subjects had clinical evidence of both caries and periodontal pathology affecting third molars. Twenty-one percent of subjects were free of periodontal pathology or caries experience.

The risk factors for periodontal disease and third-molar caries were assessed using data taken from a subset of the Piedmont 65+ study, including 340 subjects with at least one visible third molar examined for caries.[20] At enrollment, pocket depth measures were taken for 277 of the subjects. All visible teeth were examined. Pocket depth measures were taken at mesiobuccal and buccal/facial sites. Clinical data on caries experience were gathered by tactile examination. African American subjects were more likely to have a visible third molar, periodontal pathology, and clinical attachment levels of 3 mm or more on third molars. Subjects who used tobacco were also more likely to have periodontal pathology and clinical attachment level of 3 mm or more. Caucasian subjects, subjects with education beyond high school, and subjects who had visited a dentist within the past 3 years were more likely to have third-molar coronal caries experience (actual caries detected via visual or tactile examination or the presence of a restoration).

The relationship between third molars and periodontal pathology during pregnancy was a topic of interest. Consequently, data was taken from 360 patients with a mean age of 27.3 years from the patients in the Oral Conditions and Pregnancy study.[21] A full-mouth periodontal examination was conducted at six sites per tooth for each visible tooth. This was completed at less than 26 weeks of pregnancy and within 72 hours postpartum. The primary outcome was periodontal progression between enrollment and postpartum examinations. Progression was defined as four or more probing sites with an increase in pocket depth of 2 mm or more. Primary predictors at enrollment were at least one pocket depth of 4 mm or more around third molars and the upper tertile of the number of third molar probing sites recorded as bleeding on probing. One hundred twenty-two subjects (34%) experienced periodontal progression. These subjects included 74 of 176 (42%) subjects in whom a third-molar pocket depth of 4 mm or more was detected at baseline and 48 of 184 (26%) without third-molar pocket depth of 4 mm or more. Progression was found in 40 of 77 (52%) subjects in the upper tertile of the number of third-molar probing sites experiencing bleeding on probing at enrollment compared with 82 of 203 (29%) in lower tertiles. Third-molar pocket depth of 4 mm or more at enrollment or third-molar bleeding on probing was associated with periodontal disease progression.

In another study on periodontal pathology and pregnancy, data were collected from the study on Oral Conditions and Pregnancy.[22] Examinations were conducted on 1020 patients at enrollment and 891 at postpartum. Visible third-molar data were available for 405 patients at enrollment and 360 at term. Full-mouth periodontal examinations were conducted at more than 24 weeks of pregnancy and within 72 hours of delivery. Mean pocket depths by visible tooth and by jaw were calculated at enrollment and postpartum. Subjects were categorized into three broad levels of periodontal health. The primary predictor of periodontal health was the presence or absence of a visible third molar. Mean pocket depth in the mandible or maxilla at term was considered an indicator of possible risk of systematic exposure, which increases the odds of preterm birth. At enrollment and postpartum, subjects with visible third molars were significantly more likely to have moderate or severe periodontal disease than those with no visible third molars (23.5% versus 8.5% and 18.3% versus 9.4% respectively). Mean pocket depth was significantly greater for maxillary and mandibular molars than for more anterior teeth. In both jaws, mean pocket depth tended to be progressively greater from first molars to third molars. Preterm birth and elevated serum C reactive protein at term were associated more with periodontal pathology on maxillary than on mandibular third molars.

Retain Third Molars Trial: Pericoronitis

The impact of treatment for pericoronitis was evaluated by analyzing data taken from 20 patients with all third molars who exhibited minor signs or symptoms of pericoronitis.[23] Gingival crevicular fluid and plaque samples were taken from the distal of second molars and the mesial of first molars to measure the inflammatory response and identify microorganisms present. Radiographs were taken to assess alveolar bone height on the distal of second molars and the inclination/degree of eruption of the third molar. Full-mouth periodontal probing was conducted to determine pocket depths and clinical attachment levels. Pain was assessed with Gracely verbal descriptor scales and 10-cm visual analog scales. Symptomatic third-molar sites were treated with debridement and irrigation after data collection. Data were collected 1 week later and 3 months after the removal of all third molars. Gingival crevicular fluid IL-1b levels were elevated at the distal of second molars adjacent to symptomatic third molars compared with those at asymptomatic second or third molars. Alveolar bone and clinical attachment levels on the distal of second molars were normal. After 1 week, symptoms and IL-1b levels were reduced, but microbial counts were still high. After 3 months, pain was gone and alveolar bone levels and clinical attachment levels returned to initial levels.

The impact of third-molar pain, symptoms, and swelling on quality of life was assessed using data taken from 480 patients with four third molars scheduled for removal.[24] A presurgery questionnaire was administered to assess medical/dental history, reasons for seeking third-molar removal, and sociodemographic characteristics. An Oral OHIP questionnaire was administered to measure adverse impacts on oral health–related quality of life. The primary outcome variable was the percentage of people reporting 1 or more of 12 non–pain specific OHIP items "fairly often" or "very often" during the 3 months before enrollment. One third of the patients sought third-molar surgery because of current or previous symptoms of pain or swelling. Seventeen percent reported one or more non–pain specific OHIP items. The odds of one or more impacts were 2.9 times greater for people who presented because of symptoms, 1.9 times greater for people over 24 years of age, and 2.9 times greater for people with a self-reported history of tooth loss due to pathology/trauma.

Retain Third Molars Trial: Periodontitis

The association between periodontitis and asymptomatic third molars was studied in a trial that included 329 patients 14 to 45 years of age with four asymptomatic third molars and adjacent second molars.[25] Patients were enrolled for 30 months. Full-mouth periodontal probing was conducted. This probing included third molars at six sites per tooth. Pocket depth classified at 5 mm or more was an indication of periodontal pathology. Third-molar degree of eruption and degree of angulation were compared with those of the adjacent second molar analyzed by radiograph. Radiographs were used to analyze alveolar bone levels in relation to the cementoenamel junction on the distal of second molars. Demographic data on patients were collected. Twenty-five percent (82 of 329) of enrolled patients and 34% (14 of 41) of black patients had one or more pocket depth of 5 mm or more on the distal of a second molar or around a third molar. Pocket depth of 5 mm or more was associated with periodontal attachment loss of 1 mm or more. Pocket depth of 5 mm or more was associated with periodontal attachment loss of 2 mm or more in 80 of 82 patients. A higher proportion of patients 25 or older had pocket depth of 5 mm or more on the distal of second molars or around third molars compared with patients under 25 (33% to 17%). Distals of second molars and third molars in the mandible were affected more than those in the maxilla (25% to 5%).

Data were taken from 295 patients with asymptomatic third molars to determine the microbial complexes present in the third-molar region. Subgingival plaque samples were taken from the distal of second molars.[26] Probing depths at six sites per tooth were obtained to determine periodontal status. Levels of 11 bacterial species were determined with whole chromosomal DNA probes and checkerboard DNA-DNA hybridization. Detected species were grouped into "red" or "orange" complex microorganisms based on their association with periodontitis. For patients with pocket depths of 5 mm or more with periodontal attachment loss at the distal of second molars or around third molars, 10^5 or more "orange" and "red" microorganisms were detected. For patients with pocket depths of less than 5 mm in third-molar region, "orange" and "red" microorganisms were detected at levels equal to or greater than 10^5 more frequently than anticipated for patients without periodontal disease.

Three hundred sixteen healthy patients, between 14 and 45 years of age with four asymptomatic third molars and adjacent second molars were examined to determine the relationship between pocket depths and inflammation.[27] Full-mouth periodontal probing at six sites per tooth was conducted. Gingival crevicular fluid samples were taken from the mesial of all first molars and the distal of all second molars. Evaluation occurred over a 30-month period. For pocket depths less than 5 mm, inflammation for 32% of patients was negligible, for 35% midrange, and for 33% elevated. For pocket depths of 5 mm or more, inflammation for 18% of patients was negligible, for 37% midrange, and for 45% elevated.

Data were taken from 254 patients with four asymptomatic third molars and adjacent second molars to evaluate the progression of periodontal disease in the third-molar region.[28] Patients had a minimum of two annual follow-up visits and a mean age of 27.5 years at baseline. Full-mouth periodontal probing was conducted to determine periodontal status at baseline and follow-up. Radiographs were analyzed for angulation and degree of eruption of third molars. Patients were categorized as those exhibiting 2 mm or more of change in pocket depth between baseline and follow-up in the third-molar region (distal of second or around third molar) and those exhibiting less than 2 mm of change. Fifty-nine percent of the subjects had at least one pocket depth of 4 mm or more in the third-molar region and 25% had pocket depth of 5 mm or more at enrollment. Twenty-four percent of subjects had one or more teeth that had increased pocket depth 2 mm or more in the third-molar region at follow-up. Of the subjects who had at least one pocket depth of 4 mm or more at baseline, 38% had at least one pocket depth deepen by 2 mm or more at follow-up. Three percent of those subjects with all teeth with pocket depth less than 4 mm at baseline exhibited a change of 2 mm or more.

Two hundred thirty-seven healthy patients, between age 14 and 45, with four asymptomatic third molars and adjacent second molars were analyzed to examine changes in angulation and periodontal pathology.[29] Full-mouth periodontal probing was conducted to determine periodontal status at follow-up. Radiographs were analyzed for angulation and eruption of third molars. Pocket depths of 4 mm or more in the third-molar region (distal of second or around third molar) were considered clinically important at follow-up. Median follow-up was at 2.2 years. Forty-four percent of impacted maxillary and 26% of impacted mandibular third molars changed angulation/position. One third of vertical/distal impacted third molars in both jaws and 11% of mesial/horizontal mandibular third molars erupted to the occlusal plane during follow-up from baseline. At follow-up, 11% of 125 impacted maxillary third molars and 29% of 133 impacted mandibular third molars had pocket depths of 4 mm or more. Eleven percent of 307 maxillary third molars at the occlusal plane had pocket depths of 4 mm or more.

The reliability of probing depths and the impact of third-molar periodontal pathology were assessed on 41 patients.[30] Full-mouth periodontal probing examinations were conducted at less than 24 weeks of pregnancy. Periodontal status, moderate/severe periodontal disease (15 or more sites with pocket depths of 4 mm or more), and upper quartile of extent of pocket depth for third molars alone with pocket depth of 4 mm or more were considered as possible predictors of systemic inflammation and preterm birth. Data (1020 obstetric patients) for association between oral inflammation with periodontal pathology were taken from Oral Conditions and Pregnancy study. The reliability of pocket depth within 1 mm was excellent for both third molars and non–third molars. Eighteen percent of obstetric patients delivered preterm, at less than 37 weeks. Moderate/severe periodontal disease (excluding third molars) was significantly associated with preterm birth. This was more significant when third molars were included. The deeper the third-molar pockets, the greater are the chances for preterm birth.

The relationship between inflammation and the progression of periodontal pathology was examined by evaluating 254 subjects with four asymptomatic third molars and adjacent second molars.[31] Full-mouth periodontal probing was conducted at enrollment and follow-up. Enrollment levels of gingival crevicular fluid inflammatory mediators and periodontal pathogens were assayed as indicators of the degree of inflammation. Subjects were characterized as those who did or didn't have a change of 2 mm or more in pocket depth between baseline and follow-up in the third-molar region. Statistical analysis was used to indicate relationships between baseline pocket depth, levels of periodontal pathogens, levels of gingival crevicular fluid IL-1β, and the proportion of subjects with 2-mm or more change in pocket depth versus those with change of less than 2 mm. Twenty-four percent of 254 subjects experienced changes in pocket depth in the third-molar region from baseline to follow-up. Ninety-five percent of these subjects had a baseline pocket depth of 4 mm or more. Levels of "orange" and "red" complex bacteria 10^5 or more and pocket depth of 4 mm or more were both significantly associated with a change in pocket depth of 2 mm or more.

The change in third-molar and non–third-molar pathology over time was evaluated by analyzing 195 healthy subjects with a median age at enrollment of 26.2 years and a median follow-up of 5.9 years.[32] All subjects involved in the study had four asymptomatic third molars. Full-mouth periodontal probing at six sites per tooth was conducted to determine periodontal status at baseline and at longest follow-up. The third-molar region was defined as including pocket depth for six sites around third molars and two sites on the distal of second molars. Primary outcome measures were an occurrence of pocket depth of 4 mm or more and an increase in pocket depth of at least 2 mm in the third-molar and non–third-molar regions. The proportion of subjects with at least one involved site in non–third molars increased significantly from baseline to follow-up (36% to 49%). Most of these were changes in mandibular non–third molars (33% to 48%). Of the 122 subjects with one or more sites with pocket depth of 4 mm or more at baseline in the third-molar region, the proportion of subjects with one or more involved sites in non–third molars increased significantly from baseline to follow-up (48% to 59%). This also reflected mostly changes in mandibular non–third molars (44% to 59%).

An assessment was made of changes over time in third-molar position relative to the occlusal plane and in the periodontal probing status of third molars in asymptomatic subjects who had at least one third molar below the occlusal plane at baseline and retained all third molars to follow-up.[33] Between 1998 and 2002, 146 subjects who had at least one third molar not fully erupted at baseline with at least 2-year follow-up were analyzed. At baseline and longest follow-up, full-mouth periodontal probing at six sites per tooth, including third molars, was conducted. A pocket depth greater than or equal to 4 mm in the third-molar region was considered indicative of periodontal pathology. Panoramic radiographs were analyzed to assess whether unerupted third molars erupted to the occlusal plane. To assess descriptively the influence of age and length of follow-up on the change in third-molar position and periodontal status, subjects were stratified by age at enrollment as younger (<25 years) or older (≥ 25 years) and by length of follow-up as shorter follow-up (2 to <4 years), or longer follow-up (4 or more years). Because of the small sample sizes in each stratum, analyses are limited to descriptive statistics only. The anatomic position of third molars was not static over time even if subjects were more than 25 years old. Thus, unerupted third molars should be monitored for changes in position and periodontal pathology as long as the teeth are retained.

The last study relating to periodontitis cited in this paper was conducted to assess the clinical impact of risk factors for third-molar and non–third-molar periodontal pathology over time.[34] Subjects included 195 healthy adults with four asymptomatic third molars who had a median age at enrollment of 26.2 years and a median follow-up of 5.9 years. Full-mouth periodontal probing data were gathered to determine clinical measures of possible periodontal pathology. The third-molar region was defined as including pocket depth for six sites around third molars and for two sites on the distal of second molars. The non–third-molar region was defined as all remaining probing sites. Subjects were grouped based on having all pocket depth less than 4 mm (no disease), one to three pocket depths 4 mm or more (incipient disease), or at least four pocket depths 4 mm or more (early disease). Periodontal pathogen levels and gingival crevicular fluid inflammatory mediators at baseline were assayed as risk factors for periodontal pathology. Subjects who had early disease or incipient disease in the third-molar region at baseline were significantly more likely to have an indication of periodontal pathology at follow-up in both the third-molar and non–third-molar region in comparison to those who had no disease at baseline. Thus, the presence of periodontal pathology in the third-molar region at baseline was predictive of periodontal pathology in the third-molar and non–third-molar regions at follow-up for young adults.

Retain Third Molars Trial: Occlusal Caries

Occlusal caries experience was evaluated in patients with asymptomatic third molars. Three hundred three healthy patients with four asymptomatic third molars and adjacent second molars were evaluated.[35] Patient age ranged from 14 to 45. The presence and absence of caries experience on the occlusal surface of third molars and on any surface of first and second molars was recorded during clinical and radiographic examinations. The occurrence of caries experience for younger and older subjects was compared. The association of occurrence in the maxilla and mandible as well as the association between caries experience in third molars and caries experience in first and second molars was assessed. At baseline, 28% of 303 asymptomatic patients (39% of those age 25 years or more) had at least one third molar with occlusal caries. Lower third molars were more often affected than upper. Fewer than 2% of third molars had occlusal caries if the first and second molars were caries-free.

The incidence of occlusal caries in patients who had asymptomatic third molars was also evaluated in a study comparing patients who had one or more third molars at the occlusal plane with data from baseline and from the most recent of at least two follow-up visits.[36] Two hundred eleven healthy patients, of mean age 26.6 years, with asymptomatic third molars were included. The presence or absence of caries experience on the occlusal surface of any molar was recorded during clinical and radiographic examinations. Twenty-nine percent of patients were affected by third-molar occlusal caries at baseline. This percentage increased to 33% at follow-up. Ninety-eight percent and 99% of patients with third-molar caries had caries in first and second molars respectively. Older patients had more caries in their third molars at baseline than younger (under 25 years of age) patients (43% versus 9%). Patients who were younger at baseline were more likely to develop caries in third molars at follow-up (9% versus 19%). Lower third molars were affected more often than upper third molars: 25% versus 19% at baseline and 29% versus 22% at follow-up.

The prevalence of periodontal pathology and third-molar occlusal caries was evaluated on 49 patients, of median age 20.5 years, whose third molars erupted late.[37] Teeth were considered erupted once they reached the occlusal plane. All patients had at least one third-molar below the occlusal plane at baseline that erupted by the follow-up. Visual-tactile exams were conducted to assess caries experience on the occlusal surface of third molars. Periodontal pathology was indicated by at least one pocket depth of 4 mm or more in the third-molar region. The third-molar region was defined as including pocket depth for six sites around third molars and two sites on the distal of second molars. At baseline, none of the patients had occlusal caries experience in a third molar and 51% of patients had at least one pocket depth of 4 mm or more in a third-molar region. At follow-up, 27% of the patients had occlusal caries experience in at least one erupted third molar and 61% had at least one pocket depth of 4 mm or more in a third-molar region. Twenty-nine percent had occlusal caries in at least one erupted third molar and at least one pocket depth of 4 mm or more in a third-molar region. Thirty-seven percent had no third-molar occlusal caries and pocket depths less than 4 mm in all third-molar regions. Periodontal pathology was found to be more prevalent than occlusal caries in third molars that erupted late.

AMERICAN ASSOCIATION OF ORAL AND MAXILLOFACIAL SURGEONS "WHITE PAPER ON THIRD MOLAR DATA"

In 2007, the AAOMS convened a seven-member task force to review the current literature related to third-molar therapy. In conducting the review, the task force selected from four major electronic databases—Ovid Medline, PubMed, Google Scholar, and the Cochrane Database. From this, 205 peer-reviewed publications were selected to reference the compilation of the task force's finding.[38] A synopsis of these findings follows.

Regarding the natural history of third molars, the most significant variable associated with third-molar impaction is inadequate hard-tissue space. It is possible to measure this space for eruption radiographically. Unerupted teeth can change position even beyond the third decade of life. Because no reliable way has been found to predict pathologic changes associated with impacted teeth, they should be monitored periodically through radiographs. Eruption to the occlusal plane does not ensure adequate physiologic space for good periodontal health.

When considering the periodontium, root resorption of the second molar occurs more frequently when that molar is adjacent to impacted third molars, and that frequency increases with age and with mesioangular and horizontal impactions. There is an even higher frequency of periodontal ligament disruption without root resorption. There is also a greater probability of pocket depth of 5 mm or more distal of second molars when a third molar is present, and of loss of attachment of 1 mm or more. The removal of impacted third molars may negatively impact the attachment level, pocket depth, or alveolar bone height of the distal surface of adjacent second molars. The presence of intrabony defects at the time of surgery, a large contact area between the third and second molars, and inadequate postoperative plaque control may contribute to postextraction periodontal pathology in these areas. Those with healthy preoperative periodontium were also at risk for loss of attachment or increased pocket depth after third-molar surgery. No single surgical approach to the removal of third molars (flap design, tooth sectioning, or ostectomy) will minimize the loss of periodontal attachment. Guided tissue regeneration and demineralized bone allograft may be beneficial in instances where there is evidence of significant preexisting attachment loss. Further research is needed in this area. Scaling, root planing, and plaque control have the potential to reduce postoperative loss of attachment. The presence of third molars is associated with more severe periodontal disease, progressive loss of attachment on non–third molars (second molars), and more periodontal microflora, especially putative pathogens and molecular markers of inflammation.

Regarding symptomatic second and third molars, the inflammation associated with eruption and pericoronitis is associated with pain, swelling, erythema, and, perhaps, purulence. The most common bacteria identified are α-hemolytic streptococci and the genera *Prevotella, Veillonella, Bacteroides*, and *Capnocytophaga.* Yet over 440 microorganisms have been implicated. On occasion, such infections can progress to life-threatening infections. Antimicrobial therapy and surgery are indicated.

However, the absence of symptoms does not indicate absence of disease or pathology. Pathogenic bacteria ("red" and "orange" complexes) exist in clinically significant numbers around asymptomatic third molars. Periodontal disease (pocket depth $\geq$ 4 mm) exists around asymptomatic third molars, and indicators of chronic inflammation in periodontal pockets exist in and around asymptomatic third molars. Periodontal disease progression is often asymptomatic.

When considering the effects of age on various parameters relating to third molars, symptoms (pain, swelling, discomfort from food impaction, and purulent discharge) generally increase with advancing age. Periodontal defects of third molars (and adjacent second molars) are more common with advancing age. Caries prevalence in third molars increases with advancing age. Postoperative morbidity and HRQOL indicators deteriorated with advancing age (mean age for third-molar fracture is 45 years). Germectomy may be associated with a lower incidence of periodontal defects and other morbidity.

Many practitioners feel that consideration of the third molar is a necessary component of orthodontic treatment planning. However, a recent Cochrane review concluded that there is compelling evidence that impacted wisdom teeth do not contribute to crowding of the mandibular incisors.[39] The definitive answer to this question probably requires further study.

When considering the prosthodontic treatment plan, asymptomatic third molars may erupt or change position over time, even with advancing age. The potential for the development of pathology is well documented. Yet, not all teeth under a removable prosthesis develop pathology. Increased difficulty and morbidity occur if removal is deferred until later in life. Because pathology is unpredictable, impacted third molars should be monitored with periodic clinical and radiographic examinations.

Panoramic radiography remains the standard imaging technique for evaluating third molars. Its sensitivity is fair and specificity quite high. Yet other techniques may be important for high-risk third molars. High-risk third-molar signs include:

Superimposition of inferior alveolar nerve canal and third molar
Greater than normal distance from inferior alveolar nerve to third molar
Loss of cortical lines of canal
Darkening of the third-molar root
Narrowing or diversion of inferior alveolar nerve as it passes the third molar
Dark or bifid root apex

CT and "cone-beam" technology can give valuable information regarding the high-risk impaction detected with panoramic radiography.

Partial tooth removal (coronectomy) may be indicated in cases of high-risk third molars with an absolute necessity for tooth removal. There is no standard of care for this procedure because only five legitimate papers exist in the literature. The surgeon should consider using antibiotics, performing a primary closure, protecting the lingual nerve, and removing the crown while leaving the roots in place. This procedure is not without morbidity. Second surgery is often required and the consequences of surgery are frequently root migration and lingual and inferior alveolar nerve paresthesia.

Regarding the lingual flap technique, most third molars can be removed with a buccal approach. Lingual flap reflection and use of a lingual retractor are acceptable in select situations. A retractor with a suitable size and shape (broad, curved, thin, without sharp edges) must remain subperiosteal and on bone throughout the procedure. Yet, these characteristics of the retractor may or may not make any difference.

When considering whether anything should be placed in the socket, routine application of interventions is not indicated for all subjects. Those at "high risk" for periodontal defects postoperatively (age $\geq$ 25 years, attachment level $\geq$ 3 mm, pocket depth $\geq$ 5 mm) may benefit. The use of resorbable and nonresorbable membranes and platelet-rich plasma is more effective than no intervention.

Nerve damage is infrequent, but is a real concern. Inferior alveolar nerve paresthesia has a 1% to 1.5% frequency 1 to 7 days after surgery. Persistent involvement (still present after 6 months) occurs with a frequency of 0% to 0.9% and a mean of 0.3%. Lingual nerve paresthesia occurs with a frequency of 0.4% to 1.5% 1 day after surgery, with persistent involvement occurring with a frequency of 0% to 0.5%. Regarding the long buccal nerve, there are no specific reports in the literature. The mylohyoid nerve has a paresthesia frequency as high as 1.5%. Steroids do not help with prevention or recovery. Spontaneous recovery occurs 50% to 100% of the time for both inferior and lingual nerves.

The appropriate examination for assessment of a damaged nerve begins with mapping out and photographing the area involved. Testing light touch or tactile sensation with von Frey's hairs are for evaluation of A-beta fibers and pressure receptors. Two-point discrimination is used to test larger myelinated fibers. Direction sense assesses A-alpha and A-beta fibers. Pinprick sensation (pain sensation) evaluates A-delta and C fibers. Taste with the four primary tastes—sweet, sour, salty, and bitter—is also part of the assessment. Data about accuracy or variability of these tests do not appear in the literature.

When considering nerve repair, at least 50% of cases recover spontaneously. For lingual nerve repair, 50% to 90% show some recovery. Tactile sensation tends to improve while taste tends not to. For inferior alveolar nerve repair, 55% to 92% show some recovery. Data suggest that the sooner the repair (between 4.5 and 7 months), the better the results. Yet improvement can occur with late (even 47 months) repair.

SUMMARY

Not every patient has four third molars. Some have none. Not every third molar needs to be removed. Indications for the removal of symptomatic third molars are obvious. Indications for the removal of third molars to facilitate concomitant dental or medical therapy are obvious. Asymptomatic third molars may harbor a great number and diversity of microbes that may result in significant morbidity and may contribute to systemic disease. Asymptomatic third molars may contribute to the development of periodontal defects and root resorption of second molars. Associated morbidity increases with mesioangular and horizontal impactions, as well as with advancing age. Elective removal of third molars is a safe procedure and is associated with min-imal morbidity and minimal adverse impact on the quality of life. Alveolar osteitis is the most frequent postoperative problem. Postoperative anesthesia/paresthesia is the most troublesome postoperative problem. Postoperative problems increase with ad-vancing age. Most postoperative anesthesias/paresthesias resolve. Nerve repair is a helpful adjunct for those that do not resolve. Minimal flap design is effective in reduc-ing morbidity. Systemic antibiotics may or may not help. Systemic corticosteroids re-sult in less swelling and a more positive experience without added risk. Routine postoperative clinic/office visits are not necessary. Patients prefer postoperative tele-phone follow-up. Resorbable and nonresorbable membranes and platelet-rich plasma are more effective than nothing for significant osseous defects. Topical tetracycline may improve the rate of infection and alveolar osteitis.

REFERENCES

1. Kelly JF. Parameters of care for oral and maxillofacial surgery. A guide for practice, monitoring and evaluation (AAOMS Parameters of Care-92). American Association of Oral and Maxillofacial Surgeons. J Oral Maxillofac Surg 1992; 50(7 Suppl 2):1–174.
2. Helfrick J. Parameters of care for oral and maxillofacial surgery: a guide for practice, monitoring, and evaluation (version 2.0). J Oral Maxillofac Surg 1995;(53 Supp).
3. Haug RH, editor. Parameters and pathways: clinical practice guidelines for oral and maxillofacial surgery. AAOMS ParCare 01 (Version 3.0). Philadelphia: WB Sa-unders Co; 2001.
4. Carlson E, Haug RH, editors. Parameters and pathways: clinical practice guide-lines for oral and maxillofacial surgery. AAOMS ParCare 07 (Version 4.0). New York: Elsevier Publishing; 2007.
5. Haug RH, Perrott DH, Gonzalez RM, et al. The AAOMS age-related third molar study. J Oral Maxillofac Surg 2005;63(8):1106–14.
6. Chuaung S-K, Perrott DH, Susarla SM, et al. Age as a risk factor for third molar surgery. J Oral Maxillofac Surg 2007;65(9):1685–92.
7. Conrad SM, Blakey GH, Shugars DA, et al. Patients' perception of recovery after third molar surgery. J Oral Maxillofac Surg 1999;57(11):1288–94.
8. White RP Jr, Shugars DA, Shafer DM, et al. Recovery after third molar surgery: clinical and health-related quality of life outcomes. J Oral Maxillofac Surg 2003; 61(5):535–44.
9. Phillips C, White RP Jr, Shugars DA, et al. Risk factors associated with prolonged recovery and delayed healing after third molar surgery. J Oral Maxillofac Surg 2003;61(12):1436–48.
10. Foy SP, Shugars DA, Phillips C, et al. The impact of intravenous antibiotics on health-related quality of life outcomes and clinical recovery after third molar surgery. J Oral Maxillofac Surg 2004;62(1):15–21.
11. Tiwana PS, Foy SP, Shugars DA, et al. The impact of intravenous corticosteroids with third molar surgery in patients at high risk for delayed health-related quality of life and clinical recovery. J Oral Maxillofac Surg 2005;63(1):55–62.
12. Ruvo AT, Shugars DA, White RP Jr, et al. The impact of delayed clinical healing after third molar surgery on health-related quality-of-life outcomes. J Oral Maxillofac Surg 2005;63(7):929–35.

13. Stavropoulos MF, Shugars DA, Phillips C, et al. Impact of topical minocycline with third molar surgery on clinical recovery and health-related quality of life outcomes. J Oral Maxillofac Surg 2006;64(7):1059–65.

14. Hull DJ, Shugars DA, White RP Jr, et al. Proximity of a lower third molar to the inferior alveolar canal as a predictor of delayed recovery. J Oral Maxillofac Surg 2006;64(9):1371–6.

15. Shugars DA, Gentile MA, Ahmad N, et al. Assessment of oral health–related quality of life before and after third molar surgery. J Oral Maxillofac Surg 2006;64(12): 1721–30.

16. Noori H, Hill DL, Shugars DA, et al. Third molar root development and recovery from third molar surgery. J Oral Maxillofac Surg 2007;65(4):680–5.

17. Elter JR, Cuomo CH, Offenbacher S, et al. Third molars associated with periodontal pathology in the Third National Health and Nutrition Examination Survey. J Oral Maxillofac Surg 2004;62(4):440–5.

18. Elter JR, Offenbacher S, White RP Jr, et al. Third molars associated with periodontal pathology in older Americans. J Oral Maxillofac Surg 2005;63(2):179–84.

19. Moss KL, Beck JD, Mauriello SM, et al. Third molar periodontal pathology and caries in senior adults. J Oral Maxillofac Surg 2007;65(1):103–8.

20. Moss KL, Beck JD, Mauriello SM, et al. Risk indicators for third molar caries and periodontal disease in senior adults. J Oral Maxillofac Surg 2007;65(5):958–63.

21. Moss KL, Ruvo AT, Offenbacher S, et al. Third molars and progression of periodontal pathology during pregnancy. J Oral Maxillofac Surg 2007;65(6):1065–9.

22. Moss KL, Serlo AD, Offenbacher S, et al. The oral and systemic impact of third molar periodontal pathology. J Oral Maxillofac Surg 2007;65(9):1739–45.

23. Blakey GH, White RP, Offenbacher S, et al. Clinical/biological outcomes of treatment for pericoronitis. J Oral Maxillofac Surg 1996;54(10):1150–60.

24. Slade GD, Foy SP, Shugars DA, et al. The impact of third molar symptoms, pain, and swelling on oral health–related quality of life. J Oral Maxillofac Surg 2004; 62(9):1118–24.

25. Blakey GH, Marciani RD, Haug RH, et al. Periodontal pathology associated with asymptomatic third molars. J Oral Maxillofac Surg 2002;60(11):1227–33.

26. White RP Jr, Madianos PN, Offenbacher S, et al. Microbial complexes detected in the second/third molar region in patients with asymptomatic third molars. J Oral Maxillofac Surg 2002;60(11):1234–40.

27. White RP Jr, Offenbacher S, Phillips C, et al. Inflammatory mediators and periodontitis in patients with asymptomatic third molars. J Oral Maxillofac Surg 2002;60(11):1241–5.

28. Blakey GH, Jacks MT, Offenbacher S, et al. Progression of periodontal disease in the second/third molar region in subjects with asymptomatic third molars. J Oral Maxillofac Surg 2006;64(2):189–93.

29. Nance PE, White RP, Offenbacher S, et al. Change in third molar angulation and position in young adults and follow-up periodontal pathology. J Oral Maxillofac Surg 2006;64(3):424–8.

30. Moss KL, Mauriello S, Ruvo AT, et al. Reliability of third molar probing measures and the systemic impact of third molar periodontal pathology. J Oral Maxillofac Surg 2006;64(4):652–8.

31. White RP Jr, Offenbacher S, Blakey GH, et al. Chronic oral inflammation and the progression of periodontal pathology in the third molar region. J Oral Maxillofac Surg 2006;64(6):880–5.

32. Blakey GH, Hull DJ, Haug RH, et al. Changes in third molar and nonthird molar periodontal pathology over time. J Oral Maxillofac Surg 2007;65(8):1577–83.

33. Phillips C, Norman J, Jaskola M, et al. Changes over time in position and periodontal probing status of retained third molars. J Oral Maxillofac Surg 2007; 65(10):2011–7.
34. White RP Jr, Phillips C, Hull DJ, et al. Risk markers for periodontal pathology over time in the third molar and non-third molar regions in young adults. J Oral Maxillofac Surg 2008;66(4):749–54.
35. Shugars DA, Jacks MT, White RP Jr, et al. Occlusal caries experience in patients with asymptomatic third molars. J Oral Maxillofac Surg 2004;62(8):973–9.
36. Shugars DA, Elter JR, Jacks MT, et al. Incidence of occlusal dental caries in asymptomatic third molars. J Oral Maxillofac Surg 2005;63(3):341–6.
37. Ahmad N, Gelesko S, Shugars D, et al. Caries experience and periodontal pathology in erupting third molars. J Oral Maxillofac Surg 2008;66(5):948–53.
38. Pogrel MA, Dodson TB, Swift JQ, et al. White paper on third molar surgery. Available at: www.aaoms.org/docs/third_molar_white_paper.pdf. Accessed September 3, 2008.
39. Mettes TG, Nienhuijs MEL, van der Sanden WJM, et al. Interventions for treating asymptomatic impacted wisdom teeth in adolescents and adults. Cochrane Database Syst Rev 2005;18(2):CD003879.

Evidence-Based Decision Making: Replacement of the Single Missing Tooth

Paul A. Fugazzotto, DDS

KEYWORDS

• Treatment algorithms • Augmentation • Implants

Single-tooth replacement may be effected through use of a resin-bonded fixed partial denture (RBB), a conventional fixed partial denture (FPD), a removable prosthesis, or a single implant-supported crown (SIC). The use of a removable prosthesis is excluded from consideration because the final treatment result of a removable prosthesis for replacement of a single missing tooth is considered a compromise in all situations.

Although the introduction of newer therapeutic modalities, surgical and restorative techniques, and restorative materials has significantly expanded available treatment options, a greater demand is now placed on the diagnostic and treatment planning acumen of the clinician. Mastery of available treatment techniques by the surgeon and the restorative dentist may be easily and predictably accomplished. The questions confronting each clinician are when to apply each treatment modality and how to use these therapeutic approaches to their maximum benefit for the patient.

This article focuses on the factors that should be considered when making such clinical decisions and offers a framework within which to formulate appropriate treatment algorithms.

COMPARING SUCCESS RATES OF VARIOUS SINGLE TOOTH REPLACEMENT TREATMENTS

The lack of direct comparative studies assessing treatment outcomes following the use of SICs or tooth-supported FPDs does not allow indisputable proclamations to be made regarding which therapy is most appropriately employed in such situations. Section 3 of the State of the Science of Implant Dentistry Consensus Conference (held by the Academy of Osseointegration in 2006) analyzed the available literature with the aim of answering the question, "In patients requiring single tooth replacement, what are the outcomes of implant- as compared to tooth-supported restorations?"[1] In an

25 High Street, Milton, MA 02186, USA
E-mail address: progressiveperio@aol.com

Dent Clin N Am 53 (2009) 97–129
doi:10.1016/j.cden.2008.10.001
0011-8532/08/$ – see front matter © 2009 Published by Elsevier Inc.

dental.theclinics.com

effort to assess an adequate number of published articles to draw conclusions, inclusion criteria demanded only a minimum 2-year length of study. Fifty-one articles were assessed from the implant literature and 41 articles were examined from the FPD literature. The success rate of single-implant restorations at 60 months was 95.1%. The cumulative success rate of FPD and RBB was 84.0%. When conventional FPDs were assessed independently of RBBs, however, the 60-month success rate for FPDs was 94.0%. The higher failure/complication rate noted for RBBs is in agreement with that reported by Pjetursson and colleagues[2] in 2008. These investigators conducted a meta-analysis of 93 articles and reported an estimated survival rate for RBBs of 87.7% after 5 years. Failures of RBBs were most often due to debonding or recurrent caries.

Failures of FPDs were most frequently attributed to caries, periodontal disease, and endodontic pathology. Failures of retention and abutment fracture were also noted.

Valderhaug[3] assessed the status of crowned teeth over 25 years and noted caries, endodontic involvement, and periodontics pathology as the primary causes of complications with or without tooth loss.

The principal causes of implant loss or a failing implant, as defined by Albrektsson and colleagues'[4] criteria, were failure to osseointegrate following initial insertion, progressive bone loss in the face of persistent inflammation, or mechanical overload. Other complications that did not lead to implant loss included abutment loosening/fracture and crown fracture.

Salinas and Eckert[1] noted higher failure rates in data reported in older studies. The significance of this observation is subsequently discussed.

A meta-analysis of 5- and 10-year survival rates of FPDs and SICs was performed by Pjetursson and colleagues.[5] This meta-analysis included cantilevered FPDs and implant-supported FPDs. The estimated 5-year survival rates for FPDs, cantilevered FPDs, and SICs were 93.8%, 91.4%, and 94.5%, respectively. The estimated survival rates after 10 years of function for FPDs, cantilevered FPDs, and SICs were 89.2%, 80.3%, and 89.4%, respectively.

Attempts to compare 5 and 10 years' cumulative success rates of FPDs and SICs in a tooth-bounded space are complicated by a number of factors in addition to the lack of studies performing direct comparisons between the two treatment modalities.

The assessment of older studies, which may have employed techniques and materials that differ significantly from those currently used, must be undertaken with great caution. There is no doubt that today's restorative dentist has a greater number of options available for tooth preparation techniques, restorative materials, and cementation than in the past. The field of implant therapy has evolved at least as quickly as that of restorative dentistry in general. In addition to the use of a wider variety of implant diameters, lengths and morphologies, implant surface technology has dramatically altered many of the basic tenants of implantology. The time necessary to attain osseointegration has been significantly shortened, and the initial strength of the osseointegrative bond has been dramatically increased. Most germane to this discussion is that implant success and survival rates have been reported for rough-surface implants that are significantly higher than those previously reported for their smooth-surface counterparts.[6–9] Success rates for rough-surface implants exceed those in the meta-analyses already discussed for FPDs and SICs.

Finally, the understanding of implant capabilities in the face of various load applications and inflammatory insults continues to evolve. There is no doubt that older studies often reported on implants placed in less than ideal situations because of limitations in available bone and implant sizes and morphologies, or because of a more primitive understanding of implant capabilities in various scenarios. Such considerations account, at least in part, for the lesser 5- and 10-year cumulative success rates of implants reported on in older studies, compared with studies, published within the last 3 to 4 years.

The cumulative success rates of rough-surface implants supporting single crowns are at least equal to those reported on for three-unit FPDs. The questions to be answered are when to use each treatment approach and how best to maximize treatment outcomes with each therapeutic modality.

DIAGNOSTIC REQUIREMENTS

Before the initiation of active therapy, a thorough examination must be performed, a diagnosis made, and a comprehensive interdisciplinary treatment plan formulated. A full series of high-quality radiographs must be taken. When necessary, three-dimensional images are also used. Panoramic films are not utilized because their accuracy is insufficient for providing useful information for comprehensive therapy. The components of a thorough clinical examination, including periodontal probing depths, hard and soft tissue examination, models and face-bow records, are well established and not discussed here. It is important to realize, however, that a thorough examination begins with an open discussion with the individual patient. It is crucial that the clinician determine the patient's needs and desires. In this way, treatment plans may be formulated that are in the best interest of the patient and that represent a greater value for the patient.

Before formulating a comprehensive treatment plan, all potential etiologies must be identified and assessed. In addition to systematic factors, these etiologies include periodontal disease, parafunction, caries, endodontic lesions, trauma, and so forth.

The treating clinician should always formulate an "ideal" treatment plan and present it to the patient. Appropriate and predictable treatment alternatives must also be offered to the patient, thus allowing the patient to chose the treatment option to which he or she is best suited physically, financially, and psychologically.

Clinicians who fail to incorporate regenerative and implant therapies into their treatment armamentaria are depriving their patients of predictable therapeutic possibilities that afford unique treatment outcomes in a variety of situations.

Conversely, teeth that can be predictably restored to health through reasonable means should be maintained if their retention is advantageous to the final treatment plan. Clinicians who claim to be implantologists—performing only implant therapy while ignoring periodontal and other pathologies—do a disservice to patients. Such clinicians include practitioners who perform inadequate periodontal therapy to predictably halt the disease process or who remove teeth that could be treated through predictable periodontal techniques.

ABUTMENT-TOOTH CONSIDERATIONS

When assessing the appropriateness of the use of specific teeth as abutments for a three-unit FPD, it is assumed that a comprehensive diagnosis has been made and a treatment plan has been formulated, that all dental disease in other areas of the mouth has been managed, and that a nonpathologic occlusal scheme has been created. In such a situation, the abutment teeth themselves must be assessed on a number of levels (**Box 1**).

Box 1
Abutment-tooth considerations
Overall health of the dentition
Occlusal stability
Presence of parafunction
Periodontal stability
Extent of attachment loss
Restorative margin position related to the gingival margin
Clinical crown available for preparation
Amount of tooth remaining following caries excavation
Amount of tooth remaining following preparation
Need for endodontic therapy
Ability to perform endodontic therapy
Amount of tooth remaining following endodontic therapy
Presence of adequate keratinized tissue

Periodontal Stability

Pocket depths beyond 3 mm are nonideal. Pocket depths of 5 mm or greater should be considered problematic, if not pathologic. Periodontal pockets are recognized as complicating factors in thorough patient and professional plaque control. Waerhaug[10] demonstrated that flossing and brushing are only effective to a depth of about 2.5 mm subgingivally. Beyond this depth, significant amounts of plaque remain attached to the root surface following a patient's oral hygiene procedures. Professional prophylaxis results are also compromised in the presence of deeper pockets. The failure of root planing to completely remove subgingival plaque and calculus in deeper pockets is well documented in the literature.[11-15] Through the examination of extracted teeth that had been root planed until they were judged plaque-free by all available clinical parameters, Waerhaug[10] demonstrated the correlation between pocket depth and failure to completely remove subgingival plaque. Instrumentation of pockets measuring 3 mm or less was successful (with regard to total plaque removal) in 83% of the cases. In pockets of 3 to 5 mm in depth, 61% of the teeth exhibited retained plaque after thorough root planing. When pocket depths were 5 mm or more, failure to completely remove adherent plaque was the finding 89% of the time. Tabita and colleagues[16] noted that no tooth demonstrated a plaque-free surface 14 days after thorough root planning when the pretreatment pocket depths were 4 to 6 mm, even in situations in which patients exhibited excellent supragingival plaque control. This is not the forum in which to discuss pocket elimination periodontal surgical therapy. However, care must be taken to ensure no probing depths in excess of 3 to 4 mm are present around potential abutment teeth.

Furcation involvements must also be assessed and eliminated through resection or regeneration if teeth are to be considered good candidates to serve as abutments for an FPD. Periodontally involved furcations cannot be predictably "maintained" through root planning, curettage, and repeated maintenance care sessions. In a longitudinal study of patients who refused active periodontal therapy and who underwent only continuing maintenance care, Becker and colleagues[17] reported an overall rate of tooth loss of 9.8% in the mandible and 11.4% in the maxilla. The same patients demonstrated a rate of tooth loss of 22.5% for mandibular furcated teeth and 17% for maxillary teeth with furcation involvements.

Goldman and colleagues[18] assessed tooth loss in 211 patients treated in periodontal private practices and maintained for 15 to 34 years on a 3- or 6-month recall schedule. Patients were treated with root planning, curettage, and open-flap debridement. Furcation involvements were not eliminated. The overall rate of tooth loss experienced over the course of patient care was 13.4%. However, the incidence of tooth loss of maxillary and mandibular teeth with furcation involvements was 30.7 and 24.2%, respectively. Teeth that exhibited furcation involvements were lost at a greater rate than nonfurcated teeth.

McFall[19] reported on tooth loss in 100 treated patients who had periodontal disease and were maintained for 15 years or longer following active periodontal therapy. Therapy did not eliminate furcation involvements: 11.3% of all teeth were lost over the course of observation. Maxillary teeth that demonstrated furcation involvements were lost at a rate of 22.3%. Mandibular furcated teeth were lost at a rate of 14.7%. Similar findings are repeated throughout the literature.[20-22]

A study by Fleisher and colleagues[23] underscored the inability to adequately debride a periodontally involved furcation with curettes and ultrasonic instrumentation. Fifty molars were treated through closed curettage or open-flap debridement. All teeth were treated by experienced operators. The teeth were then extracted and stained for the presence of plaque and calculus. Assessment of the extracted and stained teeth demonstrated that only 68% of the tooth surfaces facing the involved furcation were plaque- and calculus-free.

Although there is no doubt that the use of microscopy and appropriate instrumentation greatly improves on this level of efficacy of furcation debridement, the three-dimensional structure of the involved furcation remains. The net result is repopulation of this area by plaque, and re-initiation of a periodontal inflammatory lesion in the area. Such an approach "slows down" the progression of bone and attachment loss and may prove valuable in an older patient, or in one who does not wish to undergo more comprehensive therapy. Most situations, however, require therapy to be aimed at eliminating the periodontally involved furcation and providing the patient with a milieu amenable to appropriate plaque-control efforts.

The treatment approach chosen, whether it is resection, regeneration, a combination of resection and regeneration, or tooth removal and implant placement, depends upon the involved furcation morphology.

Extent of Periodontal Attachment Loss

Following comprehensive periodontal therapy, abutment teeth should demonstrate a lack of probing beyond 3 mm and no furcation involvements. When active periodontal disease has been treated, however, varying degrees of supporting bone and attachment loss will have occurred. In severe cases, the tooth demonstrates mobility due to secondary occlusal trauma, defined as the development of mobility under normal load application due to reduced periodontal support. Teeth demonstrating such mobility may be ill suited to serve as abutments for a three-unit FPD.

Restorative Margin Position Related to the Gingival Margin

Restorative margin position may also influence long-term periodontal health. Plaque accumulation at the restorative margin–tooth interface is a consistent finding in research and in clinical practice.[24-31] When this margin is subgingival, the resultant increased plaque accumulation often leads to acceleration of periodontal breakdown and recurrent caries.[31] Appropriate preparation of the periodontium for restorative dentistry, including management of supporting bone, covering soft tissues and the tooth–bone interface, has been discussed in detail.[32]

Clinical Crown Available for Preparation and the Development of Appropriate Retention/Resistance Form

A detailed discussion of related concepts and techniques may be found elsewhere.[32] It is imperative that an assessment of the need or the lack of need for such therapy is completed before determining a final course of treatment, because such an assessment has a direct bearing on the physical and financial impacts of care.

The Need for Endodontic Therapy

In addition to impacting the financial ramifications of care when the tooth in question is to serve as an abutment for an FPD, the influence of endodontic therapy on the long-term prognosis of the tooth must be considered. Can endodontic therapy be performed appropriately? Will the residual tooth structure following endodontic therapy be sufficient to withstand load application over time as an abutment for a three-unit FPD? Areas of specific concern are two rooted maxillary first bicuspids following endodontic therapy are of specific concern, because the residual tooth structure in the isthmus of the tooth may be highly prone to fracture; and the aspect of the mesial buccal root of a lower molar that faces the furcation. The ribbon shaped nature of this root also renders it highly susceptible to perforation during endodontic therapy, or fracture at the time of post preparation or insertion, or in subsequent function.

The Presence of an Adequate Band of Attached Keratinized Tissue

Although a number of studies exist that assess the ability to maintain periodontal health in the face of minimal bands of attached keratinized tissue, none of these studies takes into account the added inflammatory insult placed on the periodontium when a restorative margin is placed intrasulcularly. All restorative margins trap some degree of plaque at the restorative margin tooth interface. Therefore, it is prudent to ensure that a stable band of attached keratinized tissue is present to help afford a "fiber barrier," which, in conjunction with an attachment apparatus consisting of approximately 1 mm of connective tissue attachment and a short junction of epithelium ($\sim$1 mm or less), helps prevent the initiation and propagation of periodontal disease in the area. Such a band of attached keratinized tissue, in addition to having sufficient thickness to prevent recession in the face of inflammation, trauma, or both, must demonstrate an apico coronal dimension of at least 3 mm. In the best of situations, the aforementioned short junctional epithelium and connective tissue attachment will have a dimension of 2 mm. Therefore, it is only when a third millimeter of attached keratinized tissue is present that the aforementioned "fiber barrier" overlays the alveolar bone crest.

IMPLANT RECEPTOR SITE CONSIDERATIONS

When contemplating implant placement, a number of site-specific considerations must be assessed (**Box 2**). These considerations include not only the quantity and quality of available bone for implant placement, but also the position of such bone. When adequate bone is present to place an implant but such placement will result in a nonideal implant position/angulation from a restorative or force distribution point of view, the bone that is present must be classified as inadequate. A comprehensive patient workup must include appropriate diagnostic wax-ups, to allow assessment of ideal implant position and dimension when necessary. The role of implant length and width in long-term success is often misunderstood. The misconceptions that "longer

Box 2
Implant receptor site considerations
Overall periodontal stability
Overall restorative stability
Overall occlusal stability
Quantity of available bone
Quality of available bone
Position of available bone
Potential encroachment on virtual structures

implants are better" and that the maximum-sized implant should be placed whenever possible lead to the need for a greater degree of augmentation therapy and possible encroachment on vital structures.

THE ROLE OF IMPLANT DIMENSION IN LONG-TERM SUCCESS

Crown-to-root ratios and Ante's law are considered cornerstones of treatment planning periodontally healthy and periodontally compromised patients who require prosthetic intervention. The "normal" values for the crown-to-root ratio are 0.60 for maxillary teeth and 0.55 for mandibular teeth. It is important to realize, however, that such numbers are not an indicator of periodontal health or of the absence of periodontal attachment loss around teeth. When excessive wear has occurred and attachment loss is present, the crown-to-root ratio could still be within the normal range. Therefore, a normal crown-to-root ratio should not be interpreted as an indicator of a periodontally healthy situation.

After the introduction of osseointegrating implants to the dental community, it was assumed that longer implants would be more advantageous because they would present a greater surface area for potential osseointegration and a more favorable lever arm following force application. Such a belief seemed to be borne out in early studies documenting the use of machined-screw Brånemark implants (Waltham, Massachusetts).[33–36] It is important to realize that all these studies were performed on smooth-surface hex-topped implants.

The use of shorter implants significantly impacted the development of appropriate treatment algorithms and the delivery of care. Shorter-implant use allowed the clinician to avoid vital structures such as the sinus floor and the inferior alveolar canal. Their use also eliminated the need for augmentation therapy in many situations. Even when augmentation was still required, a simpler procedure was necessary than for placement of longer implants in the same situation. Unfortunately, the use of shorter implants, has long been viewed as a compromise in patient care.

Do the available finite element analyses and clinical studies support the use of shorter implants to attain treatment outcomes comparable to those attained using longer implants?

Lum[37] found that occlusal forces were distributed primarily to the crestal bone regardless of implant length and were well tolerated by the crestal bone. Parafunctional forces, were not well tolerated by the crestal bone, leading Lum to state that parafunctional forces must be attenuated. Lum[37] also suggested the use of wider implants and a greater number of implants in patients demonstrating a significant parafunctional habit.

Pierriesnard and colleagues[38] performed a finite element analysis on 3.75-mm wide hex-headed screw implants with lengths of 6 mm, 7 mm, 8 mm, 9 mm, 10 mm, 11 mm, and 12 mm, and found that the magnitude and distribution of bone stress was constant and independent of implant length.

Lai and colleagues[39] applied 35 newton centimeters (Ncm) of vertical load to implant cylinders and found that the greatest stress was always concentrated at the neck of the implant. Peak stress was independent of implant length, but it was inversely proportional to the extent of osseointegration.

Holmgren and colleagues[40] reported that implant length had no effect on peak stress magnitude or stress distribution. Stress was concentrated at the bone crest regardless of implant length.

Himmlova and colleagues[41] also found that the greatest force concentration upon force application was always at the bone crest.

The preponderance of finite element analyses demonstrates that peak stresses are always found at the bone–implant interface at the bone crest and are independent of implant length.

CLINICAL STUDIES

Buser and colleagues[7] demonstrated no difference in implant success rates between shorter and longer lengths in an 8-year life table analysis of 2359 titanium plasma–sprayed Straumann implants (Andover, Massachusetts).

Feldman and colleagues[42] examined 5-year survival rates of 2294 rough-surface Osteotite implants (West Palm Beach, Florida) and 2597 smooth machine-surfaced implants. The difference in cumulative success rates between shorter and longer, rough-surfaced implants was 0.7% and was not statistically significant. The difference in cumulative success rates for smooth-surface implants when assessing implant length was 2.2%, which was statistically significant. Implant surface must be considered in the decision to use shorter implants in various clinical situations.

Deporter and colleagues[43] documented the survival rates of 46 mandibular overdentures, each supported by three short Endopore implants (Toronto, Ontario, Canada). The cumulative implant survival rate 5 to 6 years post therapy was 93.4%.

A publication assessing the clinical results of 5526 Straumann implants documented the use of implants of different lengths in a variety of clinical applications.[6] The implants were followed for a minimum of 72 months in function. The mean time in function was 32 months. Implant length had no influence on the reported cumulative success rates.

Anitua and colleagues,[9] in a retrospective study examining 532 implants of between 7 and 8.5 mm in length with a diameter of 3.3 to 5.5 mm, demonstrated a cumulative survival rate of 99.2%.

Even in the face of a large number of studies supporting the high long-term success rates of shorter implants, another question remains. If the patients in the aforementioned studies were reconstructed at a reduced vertical dimension due to the severity of their oral health problems, a crown-to-"root" ratio approaching the "ideal" numbers quoted for the natural dentition would have resulted. Therefore, the influence of the crown-to-implant ratio on implant success and failure rates must be examined.

Rokni and colleagues[44] examined 199 implants that had been restored with fixed prostheses. Implant length ranged from 5 to 12 mm. The mean crown-to-implant ratio was 1.5. The implants were in function for an average of 4 years. Crown-to-implant ratio and implant length had no effect on the supporting bone levels around the implants.

Tawil and colleagues[45] assessed 262 machined-surfaced Branemark implants in function for a mean time of 53 months, and they found no relationship between crown-to-implant ratio and peri-implant bone loss or implant success/failure rates.

Blanes and colleagues,[46] in a 10-year prospective study of Straumann implants placed in the posterior maxilla, reported no influence of crown-to-implant ratio on implant success in function. A recent publication documenting long-term success of 2073 implants of 6 to 9 mm in length in various applications demonstrated a cumulative success rate of 98.1% to 99%, depending on the clinical application, over a mean time in function of 36.2 months.[47]

If shorter implants are to succeed in function, they must be employed within the parameters already discussed, including appropriate diagnosis and case workup, development of a comprehensive treatment plan, and amelioration of parafunctional forces.

In addition, appropriate regenerative therapy must be performed to determine the need or the lack of need for regenerative therapy to allow placement of an implant of ideal diameter for the tooth to be replaced (**Figs. 1–3**). It is imperative that implant diameter not be chosen by the available bone. Rather, an implant diameter should be selected that is ideal for the tooth to be replaced. After this implant diameter has been chosen, it must be positioned ideally on the model, as determined by the diagnostic wax-up/surgical stent. It is only at this point that a determination is made of whether regenerative therapy is required. Adequate bone must be present or regenerated to ensure buccal and palatal/lingual bone thickness of at least 2 mm following implant placement. Failure to provide such a thickness of bone significantly increases the chances of bone resorption and implant body exposure under function over time.

Fig. 4 demonstrates a patient who presented missing a maxillary central incisor. Flap reflection revealed a fairly atrophic residual alveolar ridge. Although adequate bone was present to allow implant placement within the remaining alveolar bone, such placement would have represented a threefold compromise. Because the alveolar ridge was deficient, a soft tissue graft would have been necessary to improve the final esthetic treatment outcome. More important, the implant would have been placed off angle and subjected to traumatic off-axis loading. Hsu and colleagues[48] assessed off-angle loading at 0°, 30° and 60° using finite element analyses. They demonstrated that, for each 30° increase in off-angle loading, stress to the crestal bone increased

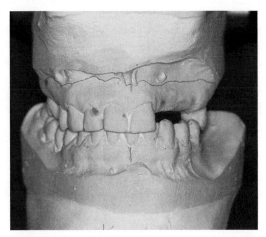

Fig.1. Face-bow mounted models demonstrate the maxillary hard and soft tissue deficiencies that must be managed if appropriate implant reconstructive therapy is to be performed.

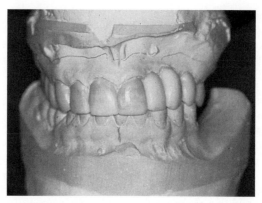

Fig. 2. A diagnostic wax-up was performed on the face-bow mounted models. The wax-up can be cut now back to the desired level so that a temporary fixed prosthesis can be fabricated, which will also serve as a regenerative guide.

three to four times. Finally, an implant of a narrower than ideal diameter would have been placed, resulting in less surface area for potential osseointegration at the bone crest, the area subjected to the greatest stresses. These stresses, in turn, would be magnified due to the off-angle loading that would occur.

To avoid these problems, appropriate regenerative therapy was performed using particulate graft material beneath a titanium-reinforced Gore-Tex membrane. The net result was an ideal ridge form that allowed placement of an implant of the desired diameter in a restoratively driven position (**Fig. 5**).

In addition to choosing implant diameter by the dimension of the tooth to be replaced, the implant chosen should demonstrate a rough surface and an internal abutment connection. The advantages of rough-surface implants as opposed to their smooth-surface counterparts have already been discussed. Meadd and colleagues[49] applied 30 Ncm of vertical and horizontal load to implants with internal or external abutment connections. Increased strain at the cervical area was noted around external abutment connection fixtures compared with internal abutment connection implants. Load also was found to be better distributed around internal connection implants than around external connection implants.

The use of wider implants has been called into question by a number of investigators. Ivanoff and colleagues[50] found a significant relationship between wider implant diameters and implant failure. Eckert and colleagues[51] found a higher failure rate of

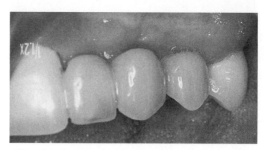

Fig. 3. Following regenerative therapy, hard and soft tissues are rebuilt to the desired levels in anticipation of implant placement and restoration.

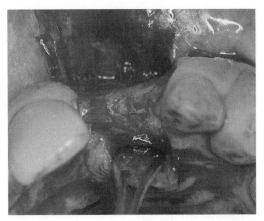

Fig. 4. A patient presented with a severely atrophic alveolar ridge in the area of a missing central incisor.

wide-diameter implants as opposed to 3.75-mm diameter implants. Shin and colleagues[52] reported a statistically significant higher failure rate of wider diameter implants compared with standard-diameter implants. However, such a finding may be due to a number of factors, including the necessary learning curve when placing wider-diameter implants and the need to minimize thermal and mechanical damage to the cortical bone during preparation. Equally important is ensurance that adequate bone will remain on the buccal and palatal/lingual aspects of the implant to attain osseointegration and maintain itself under function. As already discussed, such a concern may mandate regenerative therapy even when no implant exposure is noted following placement.

Bischof and colleagues,[53] in a 5-year life table analysis of 263 wide-neck implants, reported a cumulative success rate of 94.3% for the SICs and of 96.21% for the FPDs in the study.

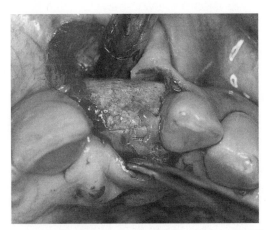

Fig. 5. The region was treated using Bio-Oss (Luitpold, Shirley, New York) and a fixated, titanium-reinforced Gore-Tex covering membrane. Note the ideal ridge form that has been attained to facilitate appropriate implant placement.

Mericske-Stern and colleagues[54] reported a 5-year cumulative survival rate of 99.1% for wide-neck implants supporting single crowns.

An implant design may also be used that is characterized by a 4.8-mm-wide body with parallel walls, which broadens to a 6.5-mm-wide platform supracrestally (**Fig. 6**). Such a design helps maintain bone buccally and palatally/lingually to the implant if the implant is placed in a ridge that has undergone resorption, atrophy, or both following tooth removal. The use of a more conventional tapered, wide-platform implant design, which begins to flare to its final restorative platform subcrestally necessitates removal of a greater amount of bone, resulting in a lesser dimension of bone buccally and lingually/palatally following placement (**Fig. 7**). Such a situation is inherently less stable under function.

When used appropriately, short implants afford a predictable means of replacing missing teeth in the least traumatic manner possible for patients (see **Fig. 6**).

UNDERSTANDING THERAPEUTIC POSSIBILITIES

Before developing treatment algorithms, it is important to be fluent in all therapeutic options for a given situation. Advances in regenerative therapy, adjunctive surgical procedures, and implant design afford the opportunity to simplify and shorten the course of therapy when faced with scenarios previously thought to be complex in nature. Three of these areas have direct bearing on the topic under discussion.

Tooth Replacement at the Time of Maxillary Molar Extraction

The ability to place an implant at the time of maxillary molar removal offers a number of advantages, including fewer surgical insults to the patient, a shorter course

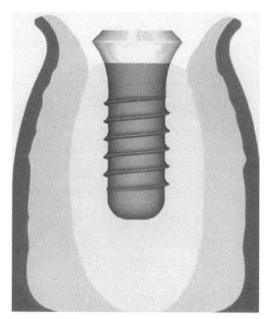

Fig. 6. Placement of a 4.8-mm-wide parallel-walled body implant with a restorative platform that expands to 6.5 mm supracrestally preserves the maximum amount of bone on the buccal and lingual/palatal aspects of the implant.

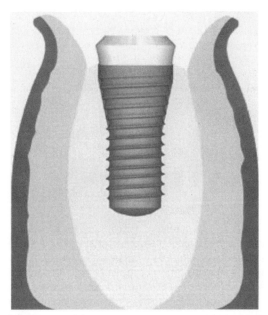

Fig. 7. Placement of a tapered implant, which begins to broaden to the final restorative platform subcrestally, results in thinner bone buccally and lingually/palatally than when using the implant design demonstrated in **Fig. 6.**

of therapy, avoidance of postextraction alveolar bone resorption and the subsequent need for regenerative therapy, and a lower overall cost of therapy. Such treatment, however, should be performed only when an ideal implant position will result.

When implant placement is to be effected at the time of maxillary molar tooth extraction, it is imperative that an implant of ideal diameter be placed in a restoratively driven position. This is easily accomplished through specific surgical techniques. It must be realized, however, that adequate interradicular bone must be present for manipulation in such a manner as to secure the implant in an ideal position following its placement. When the implant may not be so placed, augmentation must first be performed using particulate graft material and the appropriate covering membrane. The implant is placed in an ideal position following maturation of the regenerating bone **(Figs. 8–10)**.

When adequate bone is present to secure the implant in an ideal position, the implant is placed at the time of maxillary molar trisection and extraction, with or without concomitant implosion of the floor of the sinus to attain additional height for the planned implant **(Figs. 11–13)**.

A patient presented with a hopeless maxillary first molar and radiographic evidence of significant periapical pathology **(Fig. 14)**. Following tooth removal, defect debridement, and manipulation of the interradicular bone, an implant with a 4.1-mm base and a 6.5-mm-wide restorative platform was placed. Concomitant regenerative therapy was performed **(Fig. 15)**. The implant was subsequently restored with an abutment and cemented crown. After 5+ years in function, the crestal peri-implant bone is stable radiographically **(Fig. 16)**.

Using this approach, 391 implants were placed at the time of maxillary molar extraction.[55] A cumulative success rate of 99.5% was reported after a mean time in function of 30.9 months.

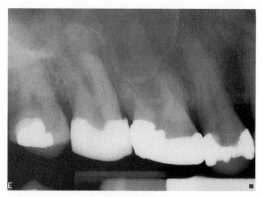

Fig. 8. A patient presented with a hopeless prognosis for a maxillary right second molar.

Figs. 17–20 demonstrate a different course of therapy. A patient presented with a hopeless maxillary left first molar and a buccal fistula that had destroyed the buccal plate of bone and a significant portion of the interradicular bone (**Fig. 17**). The tooth was extracted, the defect debrided, and the interradicular bone imploded using a previously published technique.[56] Particulate graft material and a titanium membrane were used to effect bone regeneration (**Fig. 18**). An implant was subsequently placed in the imploded and regenerated bone (**Fig. 19**). The implant has been in function for over 5 years following restoration with an abutment and crown. A radiograph demonstrates the stability of the peri-implant crestal bone (**Fig. 20**).

Implant Placement at the Time of Mandibular Molar Extraction

When adequate bone is not present to secure the appropriate-diameter implant in a restoratively driven position, augmentation is performed, and an implant is subsequently placed and restored. When sufficient interradicular bone is present, however, it may be manipulated in such a manner as to secure the implant in the desired position. Concomitant regenerative therapy is then performed, as was described for the maxillary arch. When an implant is to be placed at the time of mandibular molar extraction,

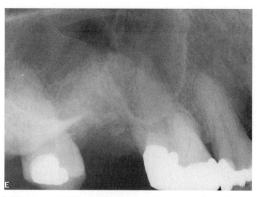

Fig. 9. Six months following tooth extraction and appropriate interradicular bone core implosion and regenerative therapy, marked bone regeneration in the extraction socket defect and preservation of the interproximal bone on the adjacent teeth are evident.

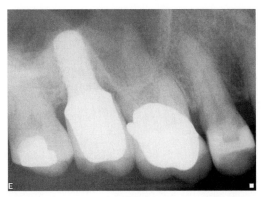

Fig. 10. A radiograph taken 5+ years after implant restoration demonstrates stable peri-implant hard tissues.

the tooth is hemisected, each root is removed individually, and any inflammatory lesions that are present are debrided. An initial osteotomy is made into the interradicular bone and a guide pin is placed (**Fig. 21**). Following the use of a differential pressure osteotomy preparation technique, a parallel-walled implant with a 4.8-mm-wide body and a 6.5-mm-wide restorative platform is placed and secured by the interradicular bone (**Fig. 22**). Concomitant regenerative therapy is performed. The implant is restored with an abutment and crown following completion of bone regeneration and osseointegration. After 5+years in function, stable peri-implant crestal bone levels are evident (**Fig. 23**).

Augmentation of the Edentulous Posterior Maxilla

Sinus augmentation therapy, with or without concomitant buccal/palatal ridge augmentation, is a highly predictable technique by which to gain adequate bone for ideal

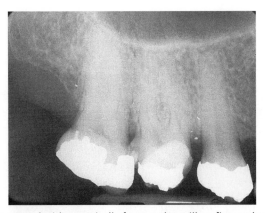

Fig. 11. A patient presented with a vertically fractured maxillary first molar. Radiographically, inadequate bone appears to be present for implant placement at the time of tooth removal. However, the radiograph shows only the bone between the buccal roots and gives no indication of the quantity of bone between the buccal roots and the palatal root.

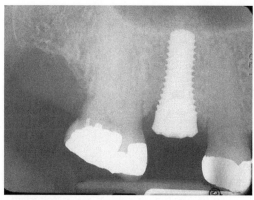

Fig. 12. A radiograph taken 6 months post interradicular bone manipulation and implosion, implant placement, and concomitant regenerative therapy demonstrates complete bone fill around the implant.

positioning of appropriate-diameter implants. However, such therapy involves a moderately invasive surgical procedure and significant protraction of the course of therapy.

In many situations, a simpler treatment alternative exists. First developed by Summers,[57] osteotomes may be used in conjunction with grafting materials to implode the floor of the sinus. This technique has proved highly predictable, within limits.

Coatoam and Krieger[58] placed 89 implants in osteotome-lifted sinuses of 77 patients and reported a 92% cumulative success rate of implants in function for 6 to 42 months. The length of the implant and implant success were not evaluated in relation to residual alveolar bone crestal to the floor of the sinus preoperatively. In addition, no effort was made to document the gain in apical alveolar bone height.

Zitzmann and Scharer[59] placed 59 implants in osteotome-lifted sinuses of 20 patients and reported a 95% cumulative success rate for the implants in function for 30 months. An apical alveolar bone height gain of 3.5 mm was reported following the osteotome procedure. The investigators stated that a minimum of 6 mm of residual

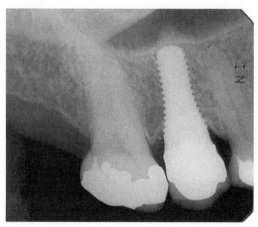

Fig. 13. A radiograph taken 7 years post restoration demonstrates stable peri-implant bone levels.

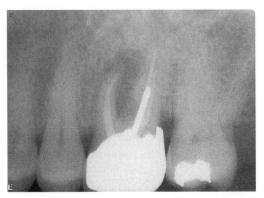

Fig. 14. A patient presented with a fistulating and hopeless maxillary first molar.

bone crestal to the floor of the sinus must be present to employ an osteotome approach with simultaneous implant placement.

Bruschi and colleagues[60] reported the results of 499 implants placed in 303 patients following the use of a localized management sinus floor technique and reported a cumulative success rate of 97% for implants in function for 2 to 5 years.

Emmerich and colleagues[61] performed a meta-analysis of sinus floor elevation using osteotomes in 2005. They concluded that the "short-term clinical success/survival ($\leq$3 years) of implants placed with an osteotome sinus floor elevation technique seems to be similar to that of implants conventionally placed in the partially edentulous maxilla."

Ferrigno and colleagues[62] reported cumulative survival and success rates of 94.8% and 90.8%, respectively, in a 12-year life table analysis of 588 implants placed at the time of osteotome use and followed for a mean observation time of 59.7 months.

It is important to realize that there are limitations to this technique. All the studies in the literature that fulfill the basic criteria of reporting at least 10 cases and of documenting the residual bone present at the time of implant placement and the length

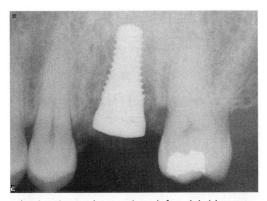

Fig. 15. Following tooth trisection and extraction, defect debridement, and manipulation of the interradicular bone, a 10-mm long tapered-end implant with a 4.1-mm-wide "apex" and a 6.5-mm-wide restorative platform is placed. Appropriate regenerative materials may now be used.

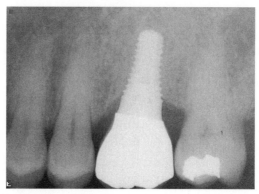

Fig. 16. A radiograph taken 38 months after implant restoration demonstrates the stability of the crestal peri-implant bone.

of implant placed demonstrate a strict correlation between implant success and residual alveolar bone height.

This correlation is especially evident in the work of Cavicchia and colleagues.[63] These investigators placed 97 implants in 86 sinuses using a modification of the osteotome approach. Eight implants were mobile at uncovery and 3 were lost in function, yielding a cumulative success rate of 88.6% after 6 to 90 months in function. Patients were treated using this approach when at least 5 mm of residual bone was present crestal to the floor of the sinus preoperatively. These investigators reported sinus displacement of 1 to 6 mm using the osteotome approach, with a mean sinus displacement of 2.9 mm apically. Six 8-mm long implants, twenty-eight 10- or 11-mm long implants, forty-seven 13-mm long implants, and sixteen 15-mm long implants were placed. Of the 8 implants mobile at uncovery, 6 were placed in patients in whom the amount of preoperative residual alveolar bone was less than 50% of the implant length. One patient demonstrated 5 to 6 mm of preoperative residual bone and had a 10-mm implant placed. Implants 13 mm in length were placed in two patients who exhibited 9 to 10 mm of preoperative alveolar bone, and a 13-mm long implant was placed in a patient who exhibited 8 mm of preoperative alveolar bone.

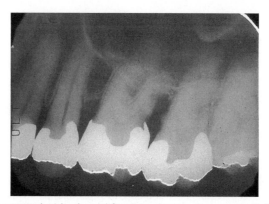

Fig. 17. A patient presented with a buccal fistula and a hopeless prognosis for a maxillary first molar. The remaining bone protecting the mesial furcation of the second molar is at risk.

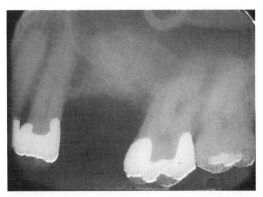

Fig.18. Six months following tooth extraction, implosion of the interradicular bone, and the use of appropriate regenerative materials, bone regeneration and preservation of the bone protecting the entrance to the mesial furcation of the second molar is evident radiographically.

A modification of the Summers[57] osteotome technique is advocated that implodes a core of alveolar bone to lift the floor of the sinus.[64] The implant is then inserted. In this manner, the implant and the graft material never touch the sinus membrane. Rather, the core of imploded bone is further displaced by the inserting implant. This core lifts the floor of the sinus, providing an "autogenous bone buffer" between the implant and the sinus floor. In addition, this core of bone supplies autogenous bone to help hasten regeneration (**Figs. 24–26**).

This technique may be used to place an implant of $2x - 2$ milimeters in length at the time of bone implosion, with x being the height of the residual alveolar bone crestal to the floor of the sinus.

A decision tree for augmentation of the posterior maxilla, whether it be by Caldwell-Luc sinus augmentation surgery, by osteotomes and trephines with or without simultaneous implant placement, or by a double osteotome and trephine technique with implant placement during the second entry, has been described.[65] It is imperative that all treating clinicians understand the capabilities of various therapeutic

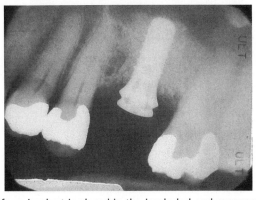

Fig. 19. A wide platform implant is placed in the imploded and regenerated bone.

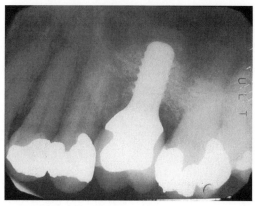

Fig. 20. A radiograph taken 8+ years in function demonstrates stable peri-implant crestal bone.

approaches. Although the restorative dentist will not perform the surgical therapies just described, he or she must be fluent in the limitations and applications of such treatment approaches to properly assess therapeutic and financial cost/benefit ratios for the patient and develop appropriate treatment algorithms.

DEVELOPING TREATMENT ALGORITHMS TO REPLACE THE SINGLE MISSING TOOTH

A number of factors must be considered when developing the most appropriate course of therapy for an individual patient. Naturally, the paramount consideration is the patient's well-being and overall health. If a patient is ill suited to be a surgical candidate, even for a minor procedure such as implant placement, such therapy should never be considered. In these situations, attempts should be made at placing a three-unit FPD.

Assuming that a patient is healthy, psychologically able to face each therapeutic option, and willing to proceed along the course of treatment suggested by the clinician, a number of factors must be assessed.

Cost of Therapy

The five primary costs of therapy are biologic, esthetic, temporal, financial, and psychologic.

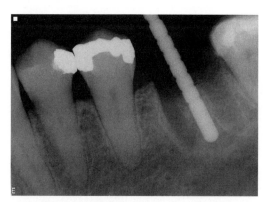

Fig. 21. Following hemisection and removal of a mandibular first molar, an osteotomy was performed in the interradicular bone and a guide pin was placed.

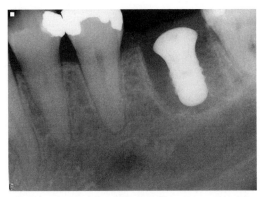

Fig. 22. A straight-walled implant with a 4.8-mm diameter and a 6.5-mm restorative platform diameter has been placed in the interradicular bone. Primary stability was attained. Regenerative therapy will now be performed.

Biologic cost

The biologic costs of maintaining a decayed tooth that requires crown lengthening include compromise of the tooth to be maintained and compromise of the adjacent teeth. Depending on the tooth preparation technique to be employed, 3 to 4 mm of tooth structure must be exposed between the alveolar crest and the planned position of the final restorative margin. In situations in which a patient presents with a short root form or with caries on the root surface, which would require removal of extensive amounts of osseous support, the tooth may be unduly compromised following crown-lengthening osseous surgery. When such a procedure would result in periodontal instability or the development of secondary occlusal trauma, crown-lengthening surgery should not be employed.

The effect of crown-lengthening osseous surgery on the entrance to a furcation of a multirooted tooth to be crown lengthened, and on an adjacent tooth, must also be considered. If attainment of an adequate amount of exposed tooth structure for restorative intervention and development of a healthy attachment apparatus results in the development of an untreatable furcation involvement, such a therapeutic approach is ill advised. Should a Class I furcation involvement result following crown-lengthening osseous surgery, it is easily eliminated through odontoplasty. Development of a furcation of any degree greater than Class I must be avoided.

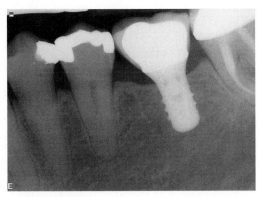

Fig. 23. A radiograph taken 54 months after implant restoration demonstrates stability of the crestal peri-implant bone.

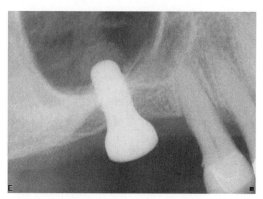

Fig. 24. A core of autogenous bone was imploded using a trephine and osteotome technique before implant placement.

Figs. 27 and **28** demonstrate two patients who presented with similar clinical problems, although their specific situations mandated different treatment approaches.

Esthetic cost

The effect of crown-lengthening osseous surgery on the patient's esthetics must be assessed. Although palatal caries on a maxillary anterior tooth may be safely exposed for restoration, the same procedure performed interproximally or buccally often results in an unacceptable esthetic treatment outcome. In such situations, other treatment options should be explored.

These same considerations must be taken into account when assessing potential abutment teeth. Just as a decayed tooth may be compromised by the necessary crown-lengthening osseous surgery or be rendered esthetically unacceptable, an abutment tooth may be at similar risk. When necessary crown-lengthening osseous surgery would cause an abutment tooth to be compromised, it should not be considered as an abutment, and an implant replacement approach should be used for the tooth that is missing.

Temporal cost

If tooth retention necessitates an excessive number of visits to perform the necessary periodontal, endodontic, and restorative therapies on the abutment teeth for the

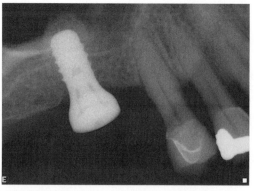

Fig. 25. Six months after bone implosion and implant placement, the autogenous bone is well consolidated around the "apex" of the implant.

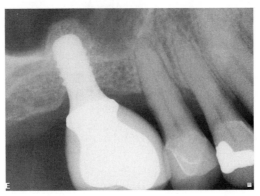

Fig. 26. After 6+ years in function, the crestal and "apical" bones around the implant are stable.

planned fixed prosthesis, the patient is often better served through implant placement and subsequent restoration. Following appropriate healing, two to three restorative visits usually is required. Such a time commitment is significantly less than that necessary when multidisciplinary treatment of abutment teeth is anticipated.

Financial cost
A recent survey polled 100 dentists in various metropolitan areas throughout the United States.[66] The costs for assorted periodontal surgical therapies, endodontic treatment of single- and multirooted teeth, posts and cores on natural teeth, tooth extraction, implant placement, implant abutments, and implant crowns were assessed relative to a given value X (**Table 1**). Such information must be taken into account by the clinician when formulating and presenting treatment options to the patient.

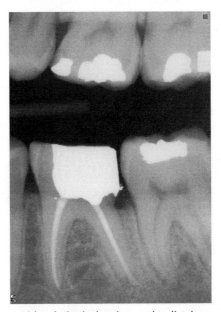

Fig. 27. A patient presents with subgingival caries on the distal aspect of a mandibular first molar. The position and extent of this caries renders the tooth an excellent candidate for crown-lengthening osseous surgery and subsequent restoration.

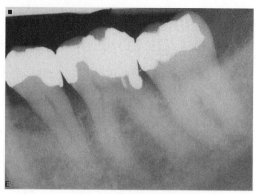

Fig. 28. A patient presents with subgingival caries on the distal aspect of a lower first molar. The extent of apical and buccal caries renders this tooth a poor candidate for crown-lengthening osseous surgery. Such a procedure would unduly compromise the second molar and would invade the buccal furcation of the first molar.

Plaque Control

The ability of the patient to perform appropriate home care efforts is crucial to the long-term success of therapy and to the selection of the appropriate treatment modality. There is no doubt that it is easier for the average patient to perform the necessary home care around an SIC than around an FPD. Although many patients demonstrate the necessary level of home care around an FPD, this treatment approach must be considered a relative hindrance to home care efforts compared with an SIC.

Retreatment Ramifications

Finally, the commitment necessary regarding retreatment must be carefully weighed by the clinician and by the patient. When the crown of an SIC fails, it necessitates

Table 1
Relative fees for various therapies

Therapy	Fee as a Factor of "X"
Endodontic—single root	0.9X
Endodontic—multiple root	1.3X
Core buildup—natural tooth	0.6X
Crown—natural tooth	1.3X
Three unit FPD	4.0X
Crown-lengthening periodontal surgery	1.1X
Regenerative periodontal surgery	1.9X
Orthodontic supereruption	2.8X
Extraction	0.3X
Implant	2.1X
Implant abutment (stock) and crown	2.2X
Implant abutment (custom) and crown	2.7X
Regenerative therapy at tooth extraction	0.7X–1.4X
Sinus augmentation	2.5X
Osteotome sinus lift	0.9X
Osteotome sinus lift at time of implant placement	no charge

Table 2
Treatment options for a single missing tooth in a tooth-bounded space

Treatment Option	Advantages	Disadvantages
Three-unit fixed bridge	Avoid implant surgical therapy Avoid vital structures Eliminate the need for regenerative therapy Slightly lesser cost of therapy than implant placement and restoration, if no endodontic therapy is required on abutment teeth	Involvement of adjacent teeth Potential for endodontic therapy Greater cost of treatment if endodontic therapy is required More difficult to perform adequate home care
Implant placement and restoration with a stock abutment and crown	No involvement of adjacent teeth Greater ease of home care Greater long-term predictability	Need to avoid vital structures Potential need for regenerative therapy Possibility of second surgical visit

replacement of the crown. Should the implant of an SIC fail, a new implant and crown are required. However, implant failure following attainment of osseointegration in a healthy patient who exhibits appropriate home care is a relatively rare occurrence.

Many clinicians advocate the use of an SIC when the teeth on either side have never been restored, citing the need to avoid involving "virgin" teeth at all costs. These same clinicians advocate use of a three-unit FPD when one or more of the adjacent teeth are heavily restored or require large restorations.

Although it is certainly logical to attempt to replace a missing tooth with an SIC if the teeth on either side have never been restored, it is illogical to cite the need for restoration of the adjacent teeth as an indication for placing a three-unit FPD. Such teeth are compromised and present with an even poorer prognosis as abutments for an FPD than previously unrestored teeth. Should one of these teeth demonstrate problems in the future, the patient would be forced to undergo more extensive, expensive treatment.

When one of the abutments of a three-unit FPD demonstrates recurrent caries, a new three-unit FPD is required. If one of the abutments fractures or becomes hopeless due to periodontal disease, a new three-unit FPD is also necessary. It also is possible that a longer-span FPD will be required, or that implant placement is necessary to effect tooth replacement in such a scenario.

Table 3
Cost analysis of treatment options for a single missing tooth in a tooth-bounded space

Treatment Option	Cost as a Factor of "X"
Three-unit fixed bridge	4.0X
Three-unit fixed bridge with endodontic therapy and buildup on one abutment	5.5X–5.9X
Three-unit fixed bridge with endodontic therapy and buildups on two abutments	7.0X–7.4X
Implant placement, stock abutment and crown	4.3X
Implant placement, regeneration, stock abutment and crown	5.0X–6.4X

Table 4
Treatment options for a missing maxillary first molar

Treatment Option	Advantages	Disadvantages
Three-unit fixed bridge	Avoid potential regenerative therapy Slightly lesser cost of therapy Significantly lesser cost of therapy if regenerative therapy is required for implant placement	Possible need for endodontic intervention Greater difficulty in plaque control efforts Potential need for periodontal surgical therapy on the second molar Second molar is often ill suited to serve as a terminal abutment
Implant placement without regenerative therapy followed by restoration with a stock abutment and crown	No involvement of adjacent teeth No need for endodontic therapy Greater ease of plaque control efforts Greater long-term predictability	Slightly higher cost of therapy than a three-unit fixed bridge without endodontic therapy
Implant placement with concomitant osteotome use, followed by restoration with a stock abutment and crown	No involvement of adjacent teeth No need for endodontic therapy Greater ease of plaque control efforts Greater long-term predictability	Slightly higher cost of therapy than a three-unit fixed bridge without endodontic therapy
Implant placement with concomitant sinus augmentation therapy, followed by restoration with a stock abutment and crown	No involvement of adjacent teeth No need for endodontic therapy Greater ease of plaque control efforts Greater long-term predictability	Greater cost of therapy than a three-unit fixed bridge without endodontic therapy
Sinus augmentation therapy followed by implant placement at a second surgical visit, followed by restoration with a stock abutment and crown	No involvement of adjacent teeth No need for endodontic therapy Greater ease of plaque control efforts Greater long-term predictability	Greater cost of therapy than a three-unit fixed bridge without endodontic therapy Need for a second surgical visit

Treatment options for replacement of a single missing tooth other than a maxillary molar in a tooth-bounded space and the cost analysis of each treatment option are presented in **Tables 2** and **3**. The cost analyses are based on the aforementioned survey of 100 practitioners throughout the United States. The financial costs of a three-unit fixed bridge or of an implant placement and restoration with a stock abutment and crown are essentially interchangeable. However, the biologic advantages of implant use in such an area, as already discussed, are significant.

Table 5
Cost analysis of treatment options for a missing maxillary first molar

Treatment Option	Cost as a Factor of "X"
Three-unit fixed bridge	4.0X
Three-unit fixed bridge with crown lengthening surgery	5.1X
Three-unit fixed bridge with one endodontic therapy	4.9X–5.3X
Three-unit fixed bridge with two endodontic therapies	6.2X
Implant placement and restoration with a stock abutment and crown	4.3X
Implant placement with concomitant osteotome therapy and restoration with a stock abutment and crown	4.3X
Implant placement with concomitant sinus augmentation therapy and restoration with a stock abutment and crown	6.8X
Osteotome therapy followed by implant placement at a second surgical visit, followed by restoration with a stock abutment and crown	5.2X
Sinus augmentation therapy with simultaneous implant placement followed by restoration with a stock abutment and crown	6.0X
Sinus augmentation therapy followed by implant placement at a second surgical visit followed by restoration with a stock abutment and crown	6.8X

When replacing a missing maxillary molar, additional considerations come into play. Sinus pneumatization may require some type of augmentation therapy. In addition, because a wide-platform implant must be used to appropriately replace a missing maxillary molar in most situations, buccal ridge augmentation therapy may also be required. The delineation of the available treatment options and the costs attendant with each option may be seen in **Tables 4** and **5**. Because of the need for Caldwell-Luc sinus augmentation therapy with concomitant implant placement or with implant placement in a second visit, which significantly protracts the course of therapy and increases the cost of treatment, care must be taken during the diagnostic phase of therapy to ensure that a simpler, less invasive approach is not feasible.

Osteotomes and trephines may often be used to effect sinus floor repositioning and augmentation before implant placement (**Figs. 29** and **30**).

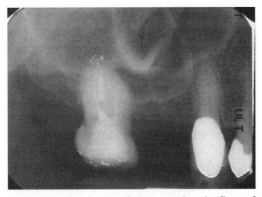

Fig. 29. A patient presented with inadequate bone crestal to the floor of the sinus for appropriate implant placement.

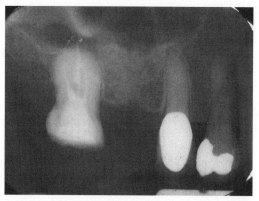

Fig. 30. Five months after an autogenous core of bone was imploded using the aforementioned trephine and osteotome technique, adequate bone is present for appropriate implant placement.

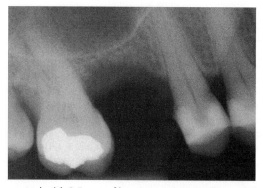

Fig. 31. A patient presented with 3.5 mm of bone crestal to the floor of the sinus. This bone is to be imploded using an osteotome and trephine technique, to a depth 1 mm less than its vertical height.

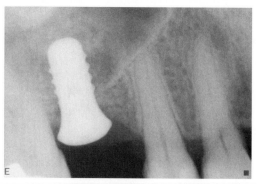

Fig. 32. Eight weeks after initial bone implosion, the developing bone is again imploded to a depth of 1 mm less than its vertical height. The implant is placed at this time.

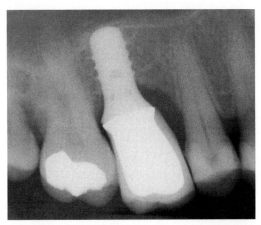

Fig. 33. Following final healing and restoration, note the level of the repositioned sinus floor and the regenerated bone in the absence of a lateral wall sinus augmentation procedure.

Even in severe cases, a double osteotome and trephine technique may often prove feasible. When a patient presents with approximately 3 to 3.5 mm of bone crestal to the floor of the sinus and adequate buccopalatal dimension for ideal positioning of an appropriate diameter implant (**Fig. 31**), an osteotome and trephine are used to implode the bone approximately 2 to 2.5 mm. Six weeks later, the newly formed bone, which now has a vertical height of 5 to 6 mm, is again imploded to a depth 1 mm less than its vertical height. An implant is placed during this visit (**Fig. 32**). The implant may be restored with an abutment and crown approximately 8 weeks after it has been inserted. **Fig. 33** demonstrates the restored implant in function for 5+ years. This therapeutic approach is significantly less invasive and less expensive than Caldwell-Luc sinus augmentation therapy followed by implant placement.

SUMMARY

Appropriate diagnosis and case workup followed by the development of a comprehensive interdisciplinary treatment plan is the cornerstone of conscientious care. Such an approach mandates an understanding of the therapeutic indications, contraindications, and possibilities of all available surgical and restorative treatment modalities. It is only in this manner that treatment algorithms may be formulated that best address individual patient needs.

REFERENCES

1. Salinas TJ, Eckert SE. In patients requiring single tooth replacement, what are the outcomes of implants as compared to tooth supported restorations? Int J Oral Maxillofac Implants 2007;22:71–92.
2. Pjetursson BE, Tan WC, Bragger U, et al. A systematic review of the survival and complication rates of resin-bonded bridges after an observation period of at least five years. Clin Oral Implants Res 2008;19:131–41.
3. Valderhaug J, Jokstad A, Ambjornsen E, et al. Assessment of the periapical and clinical status of crowned teeth over 25 years. J Dent 1997;25:97–105.

4. Albrektsson T, Zarb G, Worthington P, et al. The long-term efficacy of currently used dental implants: a review and proposed criteria of success. Int J Oral Maxillofac Implants 1986;1:11–25.
5. Pjetursson BE, Bragger U, Lang NP, et al. Comparison of survival and complication rates of tooth-supported fixed dental prostheses (FDPs) and implant-supported FDPs and single crowns (SCs). Clin Oral Implants Res 2007;18(Suppl 3):97–113.
6. Fugazzotto PA, Vlassis J, Butler B. ITI implant use in private practice: clinical results with implants followed to 72+ months in function. Int J Oral Maxillofac Implants 2004;19:408–12.
7. Buser D, Mericske-Stern R, Bernard JP, et al. Long-term evaluation of non-submerged ITI implants. Clin Oral Implants Res 1997;8:161–72.
8. Ferrigno N, Laureti M, Fanali S, et al. A long-term follow-up study of non-submerged ITI implants in the treatment of totally edentulous jaws. Clin Oral Implants Res 2002;13:260–73.
9. Anitua E, Orive G, Aguirre JJ, et al. Five-year clinical evaluation of short dental implants placed in posterior areas: a retrospective study. J Periodontol 2008;79:42–8.
10. Waerhaug J. Healing of the dento-epithelial junction following subgingival plaque control. II: as observed on extracted teeth. J Periodontol 1978;49:119–34.
11. Stambaugh RV, Dragoo M, Smith DM, et al. The limits of subgingival scaling. Int J Periodontics Restorative Dent 1981;1(5):30–42.
12. Buchanan S, Robertson P. Calculus removal by scaling/root planing with and without surgical access. J Periodontol 1987;58:159–63.
13. Jones WA, O'Leary TJ. The effectiveness of root planing in removing bacterial endotoxin from the roots of periodontally involved teeth. J Periodontol 1978;49:337–42.
14. Rabbani GM, Ash MM, Caffesse RG. The effectiveness of subgingival scaling and root planing in calculus removal. J Periodontol 1981;52:119–23.
15. Caffesse R, Sweeney PL, Smith BA. Scaling and root planning with and without periodontal flap surgery. J Clin Periodontol 1986;13:205–10.
16. Tabita PV, Bissada NF, Maybury JE. Effectiveness of supragingival plaque control on the development of subgingival plaque and gingival inflammation in patients with moderate pocket depth. J Periodontol 1981;52:88–93.
17. Becker W, Becker BE, Berg L, et al. New attachment after treatment with root isolation procedures. Report for treated class III and class II furcations and vertical osseous defects. Int J Periodontics Restorative Dent 1998;8(3):8–23.
18. Goldman MJ, Ross IF, Goteiner D. Effect of periodontal therapy on patients maintained for 15 years or longer. A retrospective study. J Periodontol 1986;57:347–53.
19. McFall WT. Tooth loss in 100 treated patients with periodontal disease—a long-term study. J Periodontol 1982;53:539–49.
20. Wood WR, Greco GW, McFall WT Jr. Tooth loss in patients with moderate periodontitis after treatment and long-term maintenance. J Periodontol 1989;60:516–20.
21. Hirschfeld L, Wasserman B. A long-term study of tooth loss in 600 treated periodontal patients. J Periodontol 1978;49:225–37.
22. Wang HL, Burgett FG, Shyr Y, et al. The influence of molar furcation involvement and mobility of future clinical periodontal attachment loss. J Periodontol 1994;65:25–9.
23. Fleischer HC, Mellonig JT, Brayer WK, et al. Scaling and root planning efficacy in multi-rooted teeth. J Periodontol 1989;60:402–9.

24. Karlsen K. Gingival reaction to dental restorations. Acta Odontol Scand 1970;28:895–9.
25. Waerhaug J. Tissue reactions around artificial crowns. J Periodontol 1953;24: 172–85.
26. Newcomb GM. The relationship between the location of subgingival crown margins and gingival inflammation. J Periodontol 1974;45:151–4.
27. Renggli HH, Regolati B. Gingival inflammation and plaque accumulation by well adapted supragingival and subgingival proximal restorations. Helv Odontol Acta 1972;16:99–101.
28. Waerhaug J. Effect of rough surfaces upon gingival tissues. J Dent Res 1956;35: 323–5.
29. Silness J. Periodontal conditions in patients treated with dental bridges. II. The influence of full and partial crowns on plaque accumulation, development of gingivitis and pocket formation. J Periodont Res 1970;5:219–24.
30. Mormann W, Regolatti B, Renggli HH. Gingival reaction to well fitted subgingival gold inlays. J Clin Periodontol 1974;1:120–5.
31. Gilmore N, Sheiham A. Overhanging dental restorations and periodontal disease. J Periodontol 1971;42:8–12.
32. Fugazzotto PA. Preparation of the periodontium for restorative dentistry. St. Louis (MO): Ishiyaku EuroAmerica, Inc.; 1989.
33. Adell R, Eriksson B, Lekholm U, et al. A long term follow-up study of osseointegrated implants in the treatment of totally edentulous jaws. Int J Oral Maxillofac Surg 1990;5:347–59.
34. Albrektsson T. A multi center report on osseointegrated oral implants. J Prosthet Dent 1988;60:75–84.
35. Fugazzotto PA, Gulbransen H, Wheeler S, et al. The use of IMZ osseo integrated implants in partially and completely edentulous patients: success and failure rates of 2,023 implant cylinders up to sixty plus months in function. Int J Oral Maxillofac Implants 1993;8:635–40.
36. Albrektsson T, Dahl E, Enbom L, et al. Osseointegrated oral implants: a Swedish multi center study of 8,139 consecutively inserted Nobelpharma implants. J Periodontol 1998;59:287–96.
37. Lum LB. A biomechanical rationale for the use of short implants. J Oral Implantol 1991;17:126–31.
38. Pierriesnard L, Reinouard F, Renoult P, et al. Influence of implant length and bicortical anchorage on implant stress distribution. Clin Implant Dent Relat Res 2003;5:254–62.
39. Lai H, Zhang F, Zhang B, et al. Influence of percentage of osseointegration on stress distribution around dental implants. Chin J Dent Res 1998;1:7–11.
40. Holmgren EP, Seckinger RJ, Kilgren LM, et al. Evaluating parameters of osseointegrated dental implants using finite element analysis: a two dimensional comparative study examining the effects of implant diameter, implant shape, and load direction. J Oral Implantol 1998;24:80–8.
41. Himmlova L, Dostalova T, Kacovsky A, et al. Influence of implant length and diameter on stress distribution: a final element analysis. J Prosthet Dent 2004;1:20–5.
42. Feldman S, Boitel N, Weng D, et al. Five year survival of short machined surface/osteotite implants. Clin Implant Dent Relat Res 2004;6:16–23.
43. Deporter D, Watson P, Pharoah M, et al. Five to six year results of prospective clinical trials using the Endopore dental implant and a mandibular overdenture. Clin Oral Implants Res 1999;10:95–102.
44. Rockni S, Todescan R, Watson P, et al. Assessment of crown to root ratios with short sintered porous surface implants. Int J Oral Maxillofac Implants 2005;20:69–76.

45. Tawil G, Aboujaoude N, Younan R. Influence of prosthetic parameters on the survival and complication rates of short implants. Int J Oral Maxillofac Implants 2006; 21:275–82.

46. Blanes RJ, Bernard JP, Blanes ZM, et al. A ten year prospective study of ITI implants in the posterior maxilla: influence of crown implant ratio. Clin Oral Implants Res 2007;18:707–14.

47. Fugazzotto PA. Shorter implants in clinical practice: rationale and treatment results. Int J Oral Maxillofac Implants 2008;23:487–96.

48. Hsu M-L, Chen F-C, Kao H-C, et al. Influence of off access loading on an anterior maxillary implant: a three dimensional finite element analysis. Int J Oral Maxillofac Implants 2007;22:301–9.

49. Meada Y, Satoh T, Sogo M. In vitro differences of stress concentrations for internal and external hex connections. J Oral Rehabil 2006;33:75–8.

50. Ivanoff CJ, Grondahl K, Sennerby L, et al. Influence of variations in implant diameters: a 3 to 5 year retrospective clinical report. Int J Oral Maxillofac Implants 1999;14:173–80.

51. Eckert SE, Meraw SJ, Weaver AL, et al. Early experience with Wide Platform Mk II implants. Part I: implant survival. Part II: evaluation of risk factors involving implant survival. Int J Oral Maxillofac Implants 2001;16:671–7.

52. Shin SW, Bryant SR, Zarb GA. A retrospective study on the treatment outcome of wide bodies implants. Int J Prosthodont 2004;17:52–8.

53. Bischof M, Nedir R, Abi Najm S, et al. A five-year life table analysis on wide neck ITI implants with prosthetic evaluation and radiographic analysis; results from private practice. Clin Oral Implants Res 2006;17:512–20.

54. Mericske-Stern R, Grutter L, Rosch R, et al. Clinical evaluation and prosthetic complications of single tooth replacements by non-submerged implants. Clin Oral Implants Res 2001;12:309–18.

55. Fugazzotto PA. Implant placement at the time of maxillary molar extraction: treatment options and reported results. J Periodontol 2008;79:216–23.

56. Fugazzotto PA. Sinus floor augmentation of the maxillary molar extraction socket: a modified technique to increase bone height. Int J Oral Maxillofac Implants 1999;14:536–42.

57. Summers RB. A new concept in maxillary implant surgery: the osteotome technique. Compend Contin Educ Dent 1994;15:152–60.

58. Coatoam GW, Krieger JT. A four-year study examining the results of indirect sinus augmentation procedures. J Oral Implantol 1997;23:117–27.

59. Zitzmann NU, Scharer P. Sinus elevation procedures in the resorbed posterior maxilla. Comparison of the crestal and lateral approaches. Oral Surg Oral Med Oral Pathol 1998;85:8–17.

60. Bruschi GB, Scipioni a, Calesini G, et al. Localized management of the sinus floor with simultaneous implant placement: a clinical report. Int J Oral Maxillofac Implants 1998;13:219–26.

61. Emmerich D, Att W, Stappert C. Sinus floor elevation using osteotomes: a systematic review and meta-analysis. J Periodontol 2005;76:1237–51.

62. Ferrigno N, Laureti M, Fanali S. Dental implants placement in conjunction with osteotome sinus floor elevation: a 12-year life-table analysis from a perspective study on 558 ITI implants. Clin Oral Implants Res 2006;17:194–205.

63. Cavicchia F, Bravi F, Petrelli G. Localized augmentation of the maxillary sinus floor through a coronal approach for the placement of implants. Int J Periodontics Restorative Dent 2001;21:475–85.

64. Fugazzotto PA. Immediate implant placement following a modified trephine/osteotome approach: success rates of 116 implants to 4 years in function. Int J Oral Maxillofac Implants 2002;73:39–44.
65. Fugazzotto PA. Augmentation of the posterior maxilla. A proposed hierarchy of treatment selection. J Periodontol 2003;74:1682–91.
66. Fugazzotto PA, Hains F. The effect of therapeutic costs on development of treatment algorithms in the partial edentulous patient. A comparative fee survey and treatment planning philosophy J Amer Dent Assoc 2008; submitted for publication.

Evidence-Based Clinical Recommendations for the Use of Pit-and-Fissure Sealants: A Report of the American Dental Association Council on Scientific Affairs

Jean Beauchamp, DDS[a], Page W. Caufield, DDS, PhD[b],
James J. Crall, DDS, ScD[c], Kevin J. Donly, DDS, MS[d,*],
Robert Feigal, DDS, PhD[e], Barbara Gooch, DMD, MPH[f],
Amid Ismail, BDS, MPH, MBA, DrPH[g], William Kohn, DDS[f],
Mark Siegal, DDS, MPH[h], Richard Simonsen, DDS, MS[i]

KEYWORDS

- Sealant • Pit-and-fissure sealant • Caries • Caries prevention
- Primary prevention • Secondary prevention
- Evidence-based dentistry • Clinical recommendations

This article was previously published in Beauchamp J, Caufield PW, Crall JJ et al. Evidence-based clinical recommendations for the use of pit-and-fissure sealants. A report of the American Dental Association Council on Scientific Affairs. JADA 2008;139(3):257–68. Copyright © 2008 American Dental Association. All rights reserved. Used with permission.

[a] 1833 Memorial Drive, Clarksville, TN 37043, USA
[b] Department of Cariology and Comprehensive Care, New York University, College of Dentistry, 345 East 4th Street, Room 1024, New York, NY 10009, USA
[c] School of Dentistry, University of California Los Angeles, 10833 LeConte Avenue, Los Angeles, CA 90095-1668, USA
[d] Department of Pediatric Dentistry, Dental School, University of Texas Health Science Center at San Antonio, 7703 Floyd Curl Drive, San Antonio, TX 78229-3900, USA
[e] Department of Preventive Sciences, University of Minnesota, 15-136 Moos Tower, 515 Delaware Street, SE, Minneapolis, MN 55455, USA
[f] Division of Oral Health, National Center for Health Promotion and Disease Prevention, Centers for Disease Control and Prevention, 4770 Buford Highway MS F-10, Atlanta, GA, USA
[g] University of Michigan, School of Dentistry, 1011 North University Avenue, D2361, Ann Arbor, MI 48109-1031, USA
[h] Ohio Department of Health, Bureau of Oral Health Services, 246 North High Street, Columbus, OH 43215, USA
[i] Midwestern University, College of Dental Medicine, 19555 N. 59th Avenue, Glendale, AZ 85308-6813, USA
* Corresponding author.
E-mail address: donly@uthscsa.edu (K.J. Donly).

Dent Clin N Am 53 (2009) 131–147
doi:10.1016/j.cden.2008.09.003
0011-8532/08/$ – see front matter © 2009 Published by Elsevier Inc.

dental.theclinics.com

Although dental sealants have been recognized as an effective approach to preventing pit-and-fissure caries in children,[1–5] clinical questions remain about the indications for placing pit-and-fissure sealants, the criteria for their placement over early caries (ie, noncavitated caries), and techniques to optimize retention and effectiveness. This report on the clinical recommendations for use of pit-and-fissure sealants presents a critical evaluation and summary of relevant scientific evidence to assist clinicians with their clinical decision-making process.

USE OF SEALANTS: AN EVIDENCE-BASED APPROACH

Dentistry is a dynamic profession, continually reshaped by new science, devices, techniques, and materials, all of which have increased rapidly since many of today's practicing dentists were trained. During the past 30 years, evidence-based approaches have developed that involve rigorous summary of findings from clinical studies about the effectiveness of preventive and treatment strategies, with the aim of providing the best available information to clinicians for decision making. In a changing practice environment, it is important that educational institutions and providers of continuing education continually update the state of the evidence related to the effectiveness of sealants in dental caries prevention and management.

Clinical decision making reflects the intersection of science, professional judgment, and patients' desires. Decisions about sealant use should be based on the best available evidence about the effectiveness of the intervention and on knowledge of the epidemiology of dental caries (risk factors and patterns of disease). Therefore, this report includes a section addressing caries' prevalence according to tooth surface and population group. This information should help to ensure that sealants are used appropriately within the context of these recommendations.

This report was developed through a critical evaluation of the collective body of published scientific evidence, conducted by an expert panel that was convened by the American Dental Association Council on Scientific Affairs. These clinical recommendations are not a standard of care, but rather a useful tool for dentists to use in making clinically sound decisions about sealant use. These clinical recommendations should be integrated with the practitioner's professional judgment and the individual patient's needs and preferences. Although these recommendations are applicable to multiple settings, the Centers for Disease Control and Prevention (CDC) is developing recommendations for use of pit-and-fissure sealants specific for school-based programs.

CARIES: DEFINITION AND PREVENTION
Definition of Dental Caries

This article defines caries as the manifestation of the stage of the caries process at any given point in time.[6] The caries process occurs across time as an interaction between biofilm (ie, dental plaque) and the tooth surface and subsurface.[6] The bacteria in biofilm are metabolically active, which causes fluctuations in plaque fluid pH. These fluctuations may cause a loss of mineral from the tooth when the pH level is dropping or a gain of mineral when it is increasing[7,8] Progression occurs when the equilibrium between demineralization and remineralization is imbalanced, leading to a net mineral loss. In clinical care settings, diagnosing caries implies determining not only whether caries is present (ie, detection) but also whether the disease is arrested or active and, if active, progressing rapidly or slowly.[7,9]

Caries is an infectious oral disease that can be arrested in its early stages. Caries can be prevented and managed in many ways. Approaches include primary prevention, defined as interventions provided to avert the onset of caries, and secondary prevention, defined as interventions to avert the progression of early caries to cavitation.

Epidemiology

In data from 2004, 42% of children and young adults aged 6 to 19 years had dental caries (decayed or filled) in their permanent teeth.[10] Prevalence of dental caries increases with age, ranging from 21% among those aged 6 to 11 years to 67% among adolescents aged 16 to 19 years.[10] The prevalence of dental caries is higher among children from low-income families and those of Mexican-American ethnicity.[10] Overall, about one quarter of carious surfaces remain untreated in children and young adults who have any caries. Approximately 90% of carious lesions are found in the pits and fissures of permanent posterior teeth.[10] These data also indicate that approximately 40% of children aged 2 to 8 years have experienced dental caries (decayed or filled) in their primary teeth.[10] Similar to findings for the permanent teeth, the prevalence of dental caries and untreated decay in the primary teeth is higher among children from low-income families and those of Mexican-American ethnicity.[10] Overall, approximately one half of carious surfaces remain untreated among children who have any caries. Approximately 44% of carious lesions in primary teeth are found on the pits and fissures of molars.[10]

The Role of Pit-and-Fissure Sealants in Primary and Secondary Prevention

Pit-and-fissure sealants can be used effectively as part of a comprehensive approach to caries prevention on an individual basis or as a public health measure for at-risk populations. Sealants are placed to prevent caries initiation and to arrest caries progression through providing a physical barrier that inhibits microorganisms and food particles from collecting in pits and fissures. It is generally accepted that the effectiveness of sealants for caries prevention depends on long-term retention.[5,11,12] Full retention of sealants can be evaluated through visual and tactile examinations. When a sealant has been lost or partially retained, it should be reapplied to ensure effectiveness.

Pit-and-fissure sealants are underused, particularly among those at high risk for experiencing caries, including children in lower-income and certain racial and ethnic groups.[13] The national oral health objectives for dental sealants, as stated in the U.S. Department of Health and Human Services initiative Healthy People 2010, includes increasing the proportion of children who have received dental sealants on their molar teeth to 50%.[14] However, national data collected from 1999 through 2002 indicated that sealant prevalence on permanent teeth among children aged 6 to 11 years was 30.5%,[15] but this represents a substantial increase over the 8% prevalence reported in a survey conducted in 1986 and 1987.[16]

Types of Sealant Materials and Placement Techniques

Two predominant types of pit-and-fissure sealant materials are available: resin-based sealants and glass ionomer cements. Available resin-based sealant materials can be polymerized by autopolymerization, photopolymerization using visible light, or a combination of the two processes.[11]

Glass ionomer cements are available in two forms, both of which contain fluoride: conventional and resin-modified.[17] Glass ionomer cements, which do not require acid etching of the tooth surface, generally are easier to place than resin-based sealants. They also are not as moisture-sensitive as their resin-based counterparts. Glass ionomer materials, which were developed for their ability to release fluoride, can bond directly with enamel. Experts hypothesize that release of fluoride from this material may contribute to caries prevention. However, the clinical effect of fluoride release from glass ionomer cement is not well established. Clinical studies have provided conflicting evidence as to whether these materials significantly prevent or inhibit caries and affect the growth of caries-associated bacteria compared with materials not containing fluoride.[18–20]

A transient amount of bisphenol-A (BPA) may be detected in the saliva of some patients immediately after initial application of certain sealants as a result of the action of salivary enzymes on bisphenol-dimethacrylate, a component of some sealant materials.[21–24] According to research, systematic BPA has not been detected as a result of the use of such sealants, and potential estrogenicity at such low levels of exposure has not been documented.[22]

Pit-and-fissure sealant materials vary, as do the techniques used to place them. Manufacturers' instructions for effective placement and long-term retention of resin-based sealants typically include cleaning pits and fissures, appropriately acid etching surfaces, and maintaining a dry field uncontaminated by saliva until the sealant is placed and cured. Supplemental techniques and recommendations as cited in the literature may include using bonding agents; using various forms of mechanical enamel preparation, such as air abrasion and modification with a bur (enameloplasty); and using the four-handed application technique.

Bonding agents, also known as adhesives, may be used when applying pit-and-fissure sealants. Current bonding systems are marketed as total- and self-etch systems. The total-etch systems involve a three- or two-step placement technique, with a separate step for acid etching. The self-etch systems are packaged either as self-etching primers with separate adhesives or all-in-one systems that combine acid etchants, primers, and adhesives. Both systems are available in single or multiple bottles.[25]

Clinical Questions Regarding Pit-and-Fissure Sealants

Although the scientific evidence supports the use of pit-and-fissure sealants as an effective caries-preventive measure, clinical questions remain about the indications for placing pit-and-fissure sealants, criteria for their placement over early (noncavitated) caries and techniques to optimize retention and caries prevention. To address these topics, the expert panel considered the following clinical questions:

Under what circumstances should sealants be placed to prevent caries?
Does placing sealants over early (noncavitated) lesions prevent progression of the lesions?
Do conditions exist that favor the placement of resin-based versus glass ionomer cement sealants in terms of retention or caries prevention?
Are any techniques available that could improve sealants' retention and effectiveness in caries prevention?

These clinical recommendations do not address the cost-effectiveness of using pit-and-fissure sealants. However, multiple models have shown that basing selection criteria for sealant placement on caries risk is cost-effective.[26,27] Readers are referred to resources cited in the reference list for further discussion of cost-effectiveness.[26–33]

METHODS

This article provides an abbreviated description of the review method used. The full methods, including the complete search strategy, are provided as Appendix 1 in supplemental data to the online version of this article (http://jada.ada.org).

The American Dental Association (ADA) Council on Scientific Affairs convened a panel of experts to evaluate the systematic reviews and clinical trials identified by staff of the ADA Center for Evidence-based Dentistry (CEBD). The council selected panelists based on their expertise in the relevant subject matter. The expert panel convened at a workshop held at the ADA Headquarters in Chicago, November 13 to 15, 2006, to evaluate the collective evidence and develop evidence-based clinical recommendations for use of pit-and-fissure sealants.

CEBD staff members searched MEDLINE to identify systematic reviews that addressed the four clinical questions.[2,5,34–42] They conducted a second search to identify clinical studies published since the identified systematic reviews were conducted.[17,33,43–78]

Members of the expert panel (Drs. Gooch and Kohn) presented a manuscript that examined individual studies included in three recent systematic reviews regarding sealant effectiveness.[2,5,79,80] CDC completed a multivariate analysis of factors associated with sealant retention, including use of the two-handed method versus the four-handed method. The included studies evaluated the retention of second- or third- generation resin-based sealant materials and provided data on whether the sealant was applied with the two- or the four-handed method.[80]

For each identified systematic review and clinical study, the panel determined the final exclusion of publications. They excluded publications based on the following criteria: they did not directly address one of the identified clinical questions; the sealant materials they described were not available in the United States; and the panelists had concerns about the methodology described. Appendix 2 in the supplemental data online is a list of excluded publications (http://jada.ada.org).

For each included publication, the panel developed an evidence statement and graded it according to a system modified from that of Shekelle and colleagues (**Table 1**).[81] The panel developed clinical recommendations based on the evidence statements. They classified clinical recommendations according to the strength of the evidence that forms the basis for the recommendation, again using a system modified from that of Shekelle and colleagues (**Table 2**).[81] Although the classification of the recommendation may not directly reflect the importance of the recommendation, it does reflect the quality of scientific evidence that supports the recommendation.

Table 1	
System used for grading the evidence	
Grade	**Category of Evidence**
Ia	Evidence from systematic reviews of randomized controlled trials
Ib	Evidence from at least one randomized controlled trial
IIa	Evidence from at least one controlled study without randomization
IIb	Evidence from at least one other type of quasi-experimental study, such as time series analysis or studies in which the unit of analysis is not the individual
III	Evidence from nonexperimental descriptive studies, such as comparative studies, correlation studies, cohort studies and case-control studies
IV	Evidence from expert committee reports or opinions or clinical experience of respected authorities

Adapted from Shekelle PG, Woolf SH, Eccles M, et al. Clinical guidelines: developing guidelines. BMJ 1999;381(7183):595; with permission.

Table 2	
System used for classifying the strength of the recommendations	
Classification	Strength of Recommendations
A	Directly based on category I evidence
B	Directly based on category II evidence or extrapolated recommendation from category I evidence
C	Directly based on category III evidence or extrapolated recommendation from category I or II evidence
D	Directly based on category IV evidence or extrapolated recommendation from category I, II or III evidence

Adapted from Shekelle PG, Woolf SH, Eccles M, et al. Clinical guidelines: developing guidelines. BMJ 1999;381(7183):595; with permission.

Because the effectiveness of sealants depends on clinical retention,[5,11,12] the panelists chose to accept clinical sealant retention as a reasonable proxy for caries prevention.

The panel submitted these clinical recommendations to numerous scientific experts and organizations for review. The expert panel scrutinized all comments received and made appropriate revisions in the recommendations. Appendix 3 in the supplemental data online provides a list of external reviewers (http://jada.ada.org). The final clinical recommendations were approved by the ADA Council on Scientific Affairs.

PANEL CONCLUSIONS BASED ON THE EVIDENCE
Evidence Regarding Sealants for Caries Prevention

Placement of resin-based sealants on the permanent molars of children and adolescents is effective for caries reduction >(see **Table 1**).[5] Reduction of caries incidence in children and adolescents after placement of resin-based sealants ranges from 86% at 1 year to 78.6% at 2 years and 58.6% at 4 years (see **Table 1**).[2,5] Sealants are effective in reducing occlusal caries incidence in permanent first molars of children, with caries reductions of 76.3% at 4 years, when sealants were reapplied as needed. Caries reduction was 65% at 9 years from initial treatment, with no reapplication during the last 5 years (see **Table 1**).[47] Pit-and-fissure sealants are retained on primary molars at a rate of 74.0% to 96.3% at 1 year [59] and 70.6% to 76.5% at 2.8 years (see **Table 1**).[59,61]

Evidence from private dental insurance and Medicaid databases consistently shows that placement of sealants on first and second permanent molars in children and adolescents is associated with reductions in the subsequent provision of restorative services (see **Table 1**).[33,66] Evidence from Medicaid claims data for children who were continuously enrolled for 4 years indicates that sealed permanent molars are less likely to receive restorative treatment, that the time between receiving sealants and receiving restorative treatment is greater, and that the restorations were less extensive than those in permanent molars that were unsealed (see **Table 1**).[46]

Evidence Regarding Placing Sealants Over Early (Noncavitated) Lesions

Placement of pit-and-fissure sealants significantly reduces the percentage of noncavitated carious lesions that progress in children, adolescents, and young adults for as long as 5 years after sealant placement, compared with unsealed teeth (see **Table 1**).[82] No findings suggest that bacteria increase under sealants. When placed over existing caries, sealants lower the number of viable bacteria by at least 100-fold and reduce the number of lesions with any viable bacteria by 50% (see **Table 1**).[83]

Evidence Regarding Sealant Materials

Results in two of three reviewed studies indicate that resin-based sealants are more effective in reducing caries at 24 to 44 months after placement compared with glass ionomer cement in permanent teeth of children and adolescents (see **Table 1**).[5,65,84,85] Limited and conflicting evidence shows that glass ionomer cement reduces caries incidence in permanent teeth of children (see **Table 1**),[17,50,51,55,65] although retention rates of glass ionomer cement are low (see **Table 1**).[5] In a population with a low caries incidence, use of glass ionomer cement is not effective in reducing the incidence of caries when placed in caries-free first primary molars (see **Table 1**).[48]

Evidence Regarding Sealant Placement Techniques

Limited and inconclusive evidence favors using air abrasion as a cleaning method before acid etching to improve sealant retention (see **Table 1**).[57] Using air abrasion instead of acid etching reduces the rate of sealant retention (see **Table 1**).[74,75] Limited and conflicting evidence shows that mechanical preparation with a bur results in higher retention rates in children (see **Table 1**).[72,73,77] Indirect evidence shows that use of the four-handed technique when placing resin-based sealants is associated with improved retention rates (see **Table 1**).[80]

Sealant retention can be improved if the clinician applies a bonding agent that contains both an adhesive and a primer between the previously acid-etched enamel surface and the sealant material (see **Table 1**).[67,68] Available self-etching bonding agents, which do not involve a separate etching step, provide comparable or less retention than do bonding agents that involve a separate acid-etching step (see **Table 1**).[69,70]

CLINICAL RECOMMENDATIONS

Table 3 presents evidence-based recommendations made by the expert panel for each question regarding the placement of pit-and-fissure sealants. The strength of each recommendation is assigned based on the level of evidence associated with each recommendation, as described in the Methods section. In instances in which the recommendation is extrapolated from the evidence, the strength of the recommendation is lowered to reflect the extrapolation.

After reviewing the evidence and developing the recommendations, the expert panel identified several areas, presented in **Box 1**, requiring additional research into pit-and-fissure sealants and further evidence.

The expert panel identified these topics as areas for additional research to provide a stronger evidence base for the application of pit-and-fissure sealants for caries prevention. These research topics were not arranged in order of priority.

Pit-and-Fissure Sealant Placement for Caries Prevention

Sealants should be placed on pits and fissures of children's primary teeth[59,61] and children's, adolescents', and adults' permanent teeth[2,5,33,46,47,55,66] when the provider determines that the tooth or patient is at risk for developing caries (see **Tables 1** and **2**).

Table 3
Summary of evidence-based clinical recommendations regarding pit-and-fissure sealants

Topic	Recommendation	Grade of Evidence	Strength of Recommendation
Caries prevention	Sealants should be placed in pits and fissures of children's primary teeth when it is determined that the tooth, or the patient, is at risk for developing caries[a,b]	III	D
	Sealants should be placed on pits and fissures of children's and adolescents' permanent teeth when it is determined that the tooth, or the patient, is at risk for developing caries[a,b]	Ia	B
	Sealants should be placed on pits and fissures of adults' permanent teeth when it is determined that the tooth, or the patient, is at risk for developing caries[a,b]	Ia	D
Noncavitated carious lesions[c]	Pit-and-fissure sealants should be placed on early (noncavitated) carious lesions, as defined in this document, in children, adolescents and young adults to reduce the percentage of lesions that progress[b]	Ia	B
	Pit-and fissure sealants should be placed on early (noncavitated) carious lesions, as defined in this document, in adults to reduce the percentage of lesions that progress[b]	Ia	D
Resin-based versus glass ionomer cement	Resin-based sealants are the first choice of material for dental sealants	Ia	A
	Glass ionomer cement may be used as an interim preventive agent when placement of a resin-based sealant is indicated but concerns about moisture control may compromise such placement[d]	IV	D

Placement techniques		
A compatible[d] one-bottle bonding agent, which contains both an adhesive and a primer, may be used between the previously acid-etched enamel surface and the sealant material when, in the opinion of the dental professional, the bonding agent would enhance sealant retention in the clinical situation[d]	Ib	B
Use of available self-etching bonding agents, which do not involve a separate etching step, may provide less retention than the standard acid-etching technique and is not recommended	Ib	B
Routine mechanical preparation of enamel before acid etching is not recommended	IIb	B
When possible, a four-handed technique should be used for placement of resin-based sealants	III	C
When possible, a four-handed technique should be used for placement of glass ionomer cement sealants	IV	D
The oral health care professional should monitor and reapply sealants as needed to maximize effectiveness	IV	D

The clinical recommendations in this table are a resource for dentists to use in clinical decision making. These clinical recommendations must be balanced with the practitioner's professional judgment and the individual patient's needs and preferences.

Dentists are encouraged to use caries risk assessment strategies to determine whether placement of pit-and-fissure sealants is indicated as a primary preventive measure. The risk for experiencing dental caries exists on a continuum and changes across time as risk factors change. Therefore, caries risk status should be reevaluated periodically. Manufacturers' instructions for sealant placement should be consulted and a dry field maintained during placement.

[a] Change in caries susceptibility can occur. The risk for developing dental caries exists on a continuum and changes across time as risk factors change. Therefore, clinicians should reevaluate each patient's caries risk status periodically.

[b] Clinicians should use recent radiographs, if available, in the decision-making process, but should not obtain radiographs for the sole purpose of placing sealants. Clinicians should consult the American Dental Association/U.S. Food and Drug Administration[97] guidelines regarding selection criteria for dental radiographs.

[c] "Noncavitated carious lesion" refers to pits and fissures in fully erupted teeth that may display discoloration not caused by extrinsic staining, developmental opacities, or fluorosis. The discoloration may be confined to the size of a pit or fissure or may extend to the cusp inclines surrounding a pit or fissure. The tooth surface should have no evidence of a shadow indicating dentinal caries and, if radiographs are available, they should be evaluated to determine that neither the occlusal nor the proximal surfaces have signs of dentinal caries.

[d] These clinical recommendations offer two options for situations in which moisture control, such as with a newly erupted tooth at risk for developing caries, and patient compliance, or both, are a concern. These options include use of a glass ionomer cement material or use of a compatible one-bottle bonding agent, which contains both an adhesive and a primer. Clinicians should use their expertise to determine which technique is most appropriate for an individual patient.

Box 1
Research recommendations

Preventive effectiveness and cost-effectiveness of various protocols for selecting patients and teeth for sealant placement

Systematic review of evidence from insurance databases regarding the effectiveness and potential cost-effectiveness of sealants in preventing caries

Clinical trials regarding the sealing of noncavitated and cavitated carious lesions using standardized diagnostic criteria

Clinical trials regarding the sealing of noncavitated smooth-surface lesions

Clinical trials regarding placement of sealants in adults

Clinical trials regarding placement of sealants on surfaces other than the occlusal surfaces of permanent molars, including premolars, buccal and lingual pits of molars, and cingula of anterior teeth

Effectiveness of different management options for noncavitated carious lesions

Methods to determine arrest of dentinal caries as measure of sealant effectiveness

Clinical trials regarding minimally invasive techniques to manage early caries (noncavitated) and cavitated carious lesions

Clinical methods to detect when an early (noncavitated) carious lesion is active or nonactive(ie, arrested)

Cost-effectiveness of caries-management strategies

Timing of sealant application

Clinical trials using sealants in adults

Clinical trials using sealants in primary teeth

The timing of caries initiation and subsequent progression of pit-and-fissure caries in contemporary populations of various caries-risk status

Research on sealant materials and retention

Enamel penetration of the materials used in the sealant application process

Depth of polymerization of sealant materials as it affects sealant retention

Additional studies of the factors that affect clinical retention and effectiveness of sealants

Evaluation of the effect of fissure-cleansing methods and materials, including laser use, on clinical outcomes

Effectiveness of self-etching primers in enhancing clinical sealant retention

Effectiveness of isolation techniques, including rubber-dam and four-handed technique

Evaluation of changes in retention associated with new products (eg, bonding agents)

Research and systematic reviews on the use of bonding agents to enhance sealant retention

Retention of light-cured sealants

Effect of mechanical preparation on sealant retention

Point-of-care application of guidelines

Translation of sealant guidelines into clinical practice

Pit-and-Fissure Sealant Placement Over Early (Noncavitated) Carious Lesions to Prevent Progression

Pit-and-fissure sealants should be placed on early (noncavitated) carious lesions, as defined in this article, in children, adolescents, young adults, and adults to reduce the percentage of lesions that progress (see **Tables 1** and **2**).[82]

Conditions that Favor the Placement of Resin-Based Versus Glass Ionomer Cement

Resin-based sealants are the first choice of material for dental sealants (see **Tables 1** and **2**).[5,50] Glass ionomer cement may be used as an interim preventive agent when placement of a resin-based sealant is indicated, but concerns about moisture control may compromise this placement (see **Tables 1** and **2**).[17,50,51,55,65]

Placement Techniques for Pit-and-Fissure Sealants

A compatible[1] one-bottle bonding agent, which contains both an adhesive and a primer, may be used between the previously acid-etched enamel surface and the sealant material when the dental professional believes the bonding agent would enhance sealant retention in the clinical situation (see **Tables 1** and **2**).[67,68] Use of available self-etching bonding agents, which do not involve a separate etching step, may provide less retention than the standard acid-etching technique and is not recommended (see **Tables 1** and **2**).[69,70] Routine mechanical preparation of enamel before acid etching is not recommended (see **Tables 1** and **2**).[57,72–75,77] When possible, a four-handed technique should be used to place of resin-based and glass ionomer cement sealants (see **Tables 1** and **2**).[80] Oral health care professionals should monitor and reapply sealants as needed to maximize effectiveness (see **Table 1** and **2**); they should consult the manufacturer's instructions for sealant placement and maintain a dry, isolated field during placement.

CARIES RISK

The panel encourages dentists to use caries risk assessment strategies in their practices. Multiple models have showed that basing selection criteria for sealants on the patient's caries risk is cost-effective.[26,27] It also is important to consider that the risk of experiencing dental caries exists on a continuum and changes across time as risk factors change.[86] Therefore, a patient's caries risk status should be reevaluated periodically. The panel recognizes that no single system of caries risk assessment has been shown to be valid and reliable. However, dentists can use clinical indicators to classify caries risk status to predict future caries experience. Caries risk assessment should be integrated with the practitioner's professional expertise to determine treatment options. The reader is referred to other resources for further discussion of caries risk.[87–93]

CLINICAL DETECTION OF NONCAVITATED PIT-AND-FISSURE CARIOUS LESIONS

Visual examination after cleaning and drying the tooth is sufficient to detect early noncavitated lesions in pits and fissures. The clinician should clean the tooth surface to remove debris and plaque before examining it for the presence of white demineralization lines or light yellow-brown discoloration surrounding the pit or fissure area. Noncavitated lesions also may appear as light to dark yellow–brown demineralization in

---

[1]Clinicians should consult with the manufacturer of the adhesive or sealant to determine material compatibility.

the pit or fissure. Clinicians should be aware that external stain is not equivalent to a noncavitated carious lesion.

After determining that a visibly cavitated lesion is not present, the examiner can dry the tooth surface with an air syringe to enable identification of early signs of dental caries. The use of explorers is not necessary to detect early lesions, and forceful use of a sharp explorer can damage tooth surfaces.[88,94–96] Clinicians should use recent radiographs, if available, in the decision-making process but should not obtain radiographs for the sole purpose of placing sealants. The Guide to Patient Selection for Dental Radiographs written by the ADA and the U.S. Food and Drug Administration[97] should be incorporated into the comprehensive care of the patient.

Many technologies are available that detect caries. Recent reviews suggest that these devices should be used only as adjunctive devices to assist in caries diagnosis.[98,99] These devices should serve primarily as a support tool for making preventive treatment plan decisions in conjunction with caries risk assessment, and sole reliance on these devices to detect caries may result in premature restorative intervention.[98]

SUMMARY

These evidence-based recommendations are a resource to be considered in the clinical decision-making process, which also includes the practitioner's professional judgment and the patient's needs and preferences. The recommendations address circumstances in which sealants should be placed to prevent caries, sealant placement over early (noncavitated) lesions, conditions that favor the placement of resin-based versus glass ionomer cement, and techniques to improve sealants' retention and effectiveness in caries prevention.

Pit-and-fissure sealants can be used effectively as part of a comprehensive approach to caries prevention. Although sealants have been used for primary caries prevention, current evidence indicates that sealants also are an effective secondary preventive approach when placed on early noncavitated carious lesions. Caries risk assessment is an important component in the decision-making process, and a patient's caries risk status should be reevaluated periodically.

ACKNOWLEDGMENT

This paper has been published previously in the Journal of the American Dental Association and has been reprinted with permission.

REFERENCES

1. National Institutes of Health Consensus Development Conference Statement. Dental sealants in the prevention of tooth decay. J Dent Edu 1984;48(Suppl 2): 126–31.
2. Llodra JC, Bravo M, Delgado-Rodriguez M, et al. Factors influencing the effectiveness of sealants: a meta-analysis. Community Dent Oral Epidemiol 1993; 21(5):261–8.
3. ADA Council on Access, Prevention and Interprofessional Relations; ADA Council on Scientific Affairs. Dental sealants. JADA 1997;128(4):485–8.
4. National Institute of Health Consensus Development Panel. National Institutes of Health Consensus Development Conference statement. Diagnosis and management of dental caries throughout life. JADA 2001;132(8):1153–61.

5. Ahovuo-Saloranta A, Hiiri A, Nordblad A, et al. Pit and fissure sealants for preventing dental decay in the permanent teeth of children and adolescents. Cochrane Database Syst Rev 2004;(3):CD001830.
6. Pitts NB, Stamm JW. International Consensus Workshop on Caries Clinical Trials (ICW-CCT): final consensus statements—agreeing where the evidence leads. J Dent Res 2004;83(spec. no.C):C125–8.
7. Kidd EA, Fejerskov O. What constitutes dental caries? Histopathology of carious enamel and dentin related to the action of cariogenic biofilms. J Dent Res 2004; 83(spec. no.C):C35–8.
8. Manji F, Fejerskov O, Nagelkerke NJ, et al. A random effects model for some epidemiological features of dental caries. Community Dent Oral Epidemiol 1991; 19(6):324–8.
9. Kid EA. How "clean" must a cavity be before restoration? Caries Res 2004;38(3): 305–13.
10. National Center for Health Statistics. Centers for Disease Control and Prevention. Available at: www.cdc.gov/nchs/nhanes.htm. Accessed October 2, 2007.
11. Ripa LW. Sealants revised: an update of the effectiveness of pit-and-fissure sealants. Caries Res 1993;27(Suppl 1):77–82.
12. U.S. Department of Health and Human Services. Oral health in America: a report of the surgeon general. Rockville (MD): U.S. Department of Health and Human Services, National Institute of Dental and Craniofacial Research, National Institutes of Health; 2000. p.166.
13. Centers for Disease Control and Prevention. Oral health: preventing cavities, gum disease, and tooth loss; 2007. Available at: www.cdc.gov/nccdphp/publications/aag/oh.htm. Accessed January 8, 2008.
14. U.S. Department of Health and Human Services. Healthy People 2010. Washington, DC: U.S. Department of Health and Human Services; 2000.
15. Beltrán-Aguilar ED, Barker LK, Canto MT, et al. Surveillance for dental caries, dental sealants, tooth retention, edentulism, and enamel fluorosis-United States, 1988–1994 and 1999–2002. MMWR Surveill Summ 2005;54(3):1–43.
16. Cohen LA, Horowitz AM. Community-based sealant programs in the United States: results of a survey. J Public Health Dent 1993;53(4):241–5.
17. Pardi V, Pereira AC, Mialhe FL, et al. A 5-year evaluation of two glass-ionomer cements used as fissure sealants. Community Dent Oral Epidemiol 2003;31(5):386–91.
18. Donly KJ, Segura A, Wefel JS, et al. Evaluating the effects of fluoride-releasing dental materials on adjacent interproximal caries. JADA 1999;130(6):817–25.
19. Mjör IA, Moorhead JE, Dahl JE. Reasons for replacement of restorations in permanent teeth in general dental practice. Int Dent J 2000;50(6):361–6.
20. Wiegand A, Buchalla W, Attin T. Review on fluoride-releasing restorative materials: fluoride release and uptake characteristics, antibacterial activity and influence on caries formation. Dent Mater 2007;23(3):343–62.
21. Arenholt-Bindslev D, Breinholt V, Preiss A, et al. Time-related bisphenol-A content and estrogenic activity in saliva samples collected in relation to placement of fissure sealants. Clin Oral Investig 1999;3(3):120–5.
22. Fung EY, Ewoldsen NO, St Germain HA, et al. Pharmacokinetics of bisphenol A released from a dental sealant. JADA 2000;131(1):51–8.
23. Söderholm KJ, Mariotti A. BIS-GMA-based resins in dentistry: are they safe? JADA 1999;130(2):201–9.
24. Vökel W, Colnot T, Csanády GA, et al. Metabolism and kinetics of bisphenol a in humans at low doses following oral administration. Chem Res Toxicol 2002; 15(10):1281–7.

25. ADA Council on Scientific Affairs. Bonding agents. Professional Product Review. Available at: www.ada.org/prof/resources/pubs/ppr/archives/07_winter.asp; 2006. Accessed January 15, 2008.

26. Griffin SO, Griffin PM, Gooch BF, et al. Comparing the costs of three sealant delivery strategies. J Dent Res 2002;81(9):641–5.

27. Quiñonez RB, Downs SM, Shugars D, et al. Assessing cost-effectiveness of sealant placement in children. J Public Health Dent 2005;65(2):82–9.

28. Deery C. The economic evaluation of pit and fissure sealants. Int J Paediatr Dent 1999;9(4):235–41.

29. Kervanto-Seppälä S, Lavonius E, Kerosuo E, et al. Can glass ionomer sealants be cost-effective? J Clin Dent 2000;11(1):1–3.

30. Kitchens DH. The economics of pit and fissure sealants in preventive dentistry: a review. J Contemp Dent Pract 2005;6(3):95–103.

31. Riordan PJ. Can organized dental care for children be both good and cheap? Community Dent Oral Epidemiol 1997;25(1):119–25.

32. Söderholm KJ. The impact of recent changes in the epidemiology of dental caries on guidelines for the use of dental sealants: clinical perspectives. J Public Health Dent 1995;55(5 spec. no.):302–11.

33. Weintraub JA, Stearns SC, Rozier RG, et al. Treatment outcomes and costs of dental sealants among children enrolled in Medicaid. Am J Public Health 2001; 91(11):1877–81.

34. Bader JD, Shugars DA, Bonito AJ. A systematic review of selected caries prevention and management methods. Community Dent Oral Epidemiol 2001;29(6): 399–411.

35. Bader JD, Shugars DA, Bonito AJ. Systematic reviews of selected dental caries diagnostic and management methods. J Dent Edu 2001;65(10):960–8.

36. Hiiri A, Ahovuo-Saloranta A, Nordblad A, et al. Pit and fissure sealants versus fluoride varnishes for preventing dental decay in children and adolescents. Cochrane Database Syst Rev 2006;(4):CD003067.

37. Källestål C, Norlund A, Söder B, et al. Economic evaluation of dental caries prevention: a systematic review. Acta Odontol Scand 2003;61(6):341–6.

38. Mejáre I, Lingström P, Petersson LG, et al. Caries-preventive effect of fissure sealants: a systematic review. Acta Odontol Scand 2003;61(6):321–30.

39. Muller-Bolla M, Lupi-Pégurier L, Tardieu C, et al. Retention of resin-based pit and fissure sealants: a systematic review. Community Dent Oral Epidemiol 2006; 34(5):321–36.

40. Rozier RG. Effectiveness of methods used by dental professionals for the primary prevention of dental caries. J Dent Educ 2001;65(10):1063–72.

41. Tinanoff N, Douglass JM. Clinical decision-making for caries management in primary teeth. J Dent Educ 2001;65(10):1133–42.

42. Beiruti N, Frencken JE, van't Hoff MA, et al. Caries-preventive effect of resin-based and glass ionomer sealants over time: a systematic review. Community Dent Oral Epidemiol 2006;34(6):403–9.

43. Beiruti N, Frencken JE, van't Hoff MA, et al. Caries-preventive effect of a one-time application of composite resin and glass ionomer sealants after 5 years. Caries Res 2006;40(1):52–9.

44. Albani F, Ballesio I, Campanella V, et al. Pit and fissure sealants: results at five and ten years. Eur J Paediatr Dent 2005;6(2):61–5.

45. Benteke M, Berntsson L, Broman U, et al. Population- vs. risk-based applications of fissure sealants in first permanent molars: a 13-year follow-up. Oral Health Prev Dent 2006;4(2):151–6.

46. Bhuridej P, Damiano PC, Kuthy RA, et al. Natural history of treatment outcomes of permanent first molars: a study of sealant effectiveness. JADA 2005;136(9): 1265–72.

47. Bravo M, Montero J, Bravo JJ, et al. Sealant and fluoride varnish in caries: a randomized trial. J Dent Res 2005;84(12):1138–43.

48. Chadwick BL, Treasure ET, Playle RA. A randomized controlled trial to determine the effectiveness of glass ionomer sealants in pre-school children. Caries Res 2005;39(1):34–40.

49. Lekic PC, Deng D, Brothwell D. Clinical evaluation of sealants and preventive resin restorations in a group of environmentally homogeneous children. J Dent Child (Chic) 2006;73(1):15–9.

50. Pardi V, Pereira AC, Ambrosano GM, et al. Clinical evaluation of three different materials used as pit and fissure sealant: 24-months results. J Clin Pediatr Dent 2005;29(2):133–7.

51. Pereira AC, Pardi V, Mialhe FL, et al. A 3-year clinical evaluation of glass-ionomer cements used as fissure sealants. Am J Dent 2003;16(1):23–7.

52. Pinar A, Sepet E, Aren G, et al. Clinical performance of sealants with and without a bonding agent. Quintessence Int 2005;36(5):355–60.

53. Poulsen P. Retention of glass ionomer sealant in primary teeth in young children. Eur J Paediatr Dent 2003;4(2):96–8.

54. Poulsen S, Laurberg L, Vaeth M, et al. A field trial of resin-based and glass-ionomer fissure sealants: clinical and radiographic assessment of caries. Community Dent Oral Epidemiol 2006;34(1):36–40.

55. Taifour D, Frencken JE, Van't Hof MA, et al. Effects of glass ionomer sealants in newly erupted first molars after 5 years: a pilot study. Community Dent Oral Epidemiol 2003;31(4):314–9.

56. Yakut N, Sönmez H. Resin composite sealant vs. polyacid-modified resin composite applied to post eruptive mature and immature molars: two-year clinical study. J Clin Pediatr Dent 2006;30(3):215–8.

57. Yazici AR, Kiremitçi A, Celik C, et al. A two-year clinical evaluation of pit and fissure sealants placed with and without air abrasion pretreatment in teenagers. JADA 2006;137(10):1401–5.

58. Bagramian RA, Srivastava S, Graves RC. Pattern of sealant retention in children receiving a combination of caries-preventive methods: three-year results. JADA 1979;98(1):46–50.

59. Hotuman E, Rølling I, Poulsen S. Fissure sealants in a group of 3–4 year old children. Int J Paediatr Dent 1998;8(2):159–60.

60. Li SH, Kingman A, Forthofer R, et al. Comparison of tooth surface-specific dental caries attack patterns in US schoolchildren from two national surveys. J Dent Res 1993;72(10):1398–405.

61. Hardison JR, Collier DR, Sprouse LW, et al. Retention of pit and fissure sealant on the primary molars of a 3- and 4-year old children after 1 year. JADA 1987;114(5): 613–5.

62. Jones RB. The effects for recall patients of a comprehensive sealant program in a clinical dental public health setting. J Public Health Dent 1986;46(3):152–5.

63. Richardson BA, Smith DC, Hargreaves JA. A 5-year clinical evaluation of the effectiveness of a fissure sealant in mentally retarded Canadian children. Community Dent Oral Epidemiol 1981;9(4):170–4.

64. Cline JT, Messer LB. Long term retention of sealants applied by inexperienced operators in Minneapolis. Community Dent Oral Epidemiol 1979;7(4): 206–12.

65. Songpaisan Y, Bratthall D, Phantumvanit P, et al. Effects of glass ionomer cement, resin-based pit and fissure sealant and HF applications on occlusal caries in a developing country field trial. Community Dent Oral Epidemiol 1995;23(1):25–9.

66. Dennison JB, Straffon LH, Smith RC. Effectiveness of sealant treatment over five years in an insured population. JADA 2000;131(5):597–605.

67. Feigal RJ, Musherure P, Gillespie B, et al. Improved sealant retention with bonding agents: a clinical study of two-bottle and single-bottle systems. J Dent Res 2000;79(11):1850–6.

68. Boksman L, McConnell RJ, Carson B, et al. A 2-year clinical evaluation of two pit and fissure sealants placed with and without the use of a bonding agent. Quintessence Int 1993;24(2):131–3.

69. Feigal RJ, Quelhas I. Clinical trial of a self-etching adhesive for sealant application: success at 24 months with Prompt L-Pop. Am J Dent 2003;16(4):249–51.

70. Venker DJ, Kuthy RA, Qian F, et al. Twelve-month sealant retention in a school-based program using a self-etching primer/adhesive. J Public Health Dent 2004;64(4):191–7.

71. Mascarenhas A, Nazar H, Soparkar P, et al. Effectiveness of primer and bond in sealant retention and caries prevention. Pediatr Dent 2008;30(1):500–4.

72. Shapira J, Eidelman E. The influence of mechanical preparation of enamel prior to etching on the retention of sealants. J Pedod 1982;6(4):283–7.

73. Shapira J, Eidelman E. The influence of mechanical preparation of enamel prior to etching on the retention of sealants: three-year follow-up. J Pedod 1984;8(3):272–7.

74. Kanellis MJ, Warren JJ, Levy SM. Comparison of air abrasion versus acid etch sealant techniques: six-month retention. Pediatr Dent 1997;19(4):258–61.

75. Kanellis MJ, Warren JJ, Levy SM. A comparison of sealant placement techniques and 12-month retention rates. J Public Health Dent 2000;60(1):53–6.

76. Le Bell Y, Forsten L. Sealing of preventively enlarged fissures. Acta Odontol Scand 1980;38(2):101–4.

77. Shapira J, Eidelman E. Six-year clinical evaluation of fissure sealants placed after mechanical preparation: a matched pair study. Pediatr Dent 1986;8(3):204–5.

78. Lygidakis NA, Oulis KI, Christodoulidis A. Evaluation of fissure sealants retention following four different isolation and surface preparation techniques: four years clinical trial. J Clin Pediatr Dent 1994;19(1):23–5.

79. Gooch BF, Truman BI, Griffin SO, et al. A comparison of selected evidence reviews and recommendations on interventions to prevent dental caries, oral and pharyngeal cancers, and sports-related craniofacial injuries. Am J Prev Med 2002;23(Suppl 1):55–80.

80. Griffin SO, Jones K, Gray SK, et al. Exploring four-handed delivery and retention of resin-based sealants. JADA 2008;139(3):281–9.

81. Shekelle PG, Woolf SH, Eccles M, et al. Clinical guidelines: developing guidelines. BMJ 1999;381(7183):593–6.

82. Griffin SO, Oong E, Kohn W, et al. The effectiveness of sealants in managing carious lesions. J Dent Res 2008;87(2):169–74.

83. Oong EM, Griffin SO, Kohn W, et al. The effect of dental sealants on bacteria levels in caries lesions: a review of the evidence. JADA 2008;139(3):271–8.

84. Poulsen S, Beiruti N, Sadat N. A comparison of retention and the effect on caries of fissure sealing with a glass-ionomer and a resin-based sealant. Community Dent Oral Epidemiol 2001;29(4):298–301.

85. Arrow P, Riordan PJ. Retention and caries preventive effects of a GIC and a resin-based fissure sealant. Community Dent Oral Epidemiol 1995;23(5):282–5.

86. Recommendations for using fluoride to prevent and control dental caries in the United States. Centers for disease control and prevention. MMWR Recomm Rep 2001;50(RR-14):1–42.
87. American Academy of Pediatric Dentistry. Council on Clinical Affairs. Policy on the use of a caries-risk assessment tool (CAT) for infants, children, and adolescents. In: American Academy of Pediatric Dentistry. Reference manual 2002–2003. Chicago: American Academy of Pediatric Dentistry; 2002.
88. American Dental Association, Council on Access, Prevention and Interprofessional Relations. Caries diagnosis and risk assessment: a review of preventive strategies and management. JADA 1995;126(Suppl):1S–24S.
89. Bader JD, Perrin NA, Maupomé G, et al. Validation of a simple approach to caries risk assessment. J Public Health Dent 2005;65(2):76–81.
90. Featherstone JD. The caries balance: the basis for caries management by risk assessment. Oral Health Prev Dent 2004;2(Suppl 1):259–64.
91. Featherstone JD, Adair SM, Anderson MH, et al. Caries management by risk assessment by risk assessment: consensus statement, April 2002. J Calif Dent Assoc 2003;31(3):257–69.
92. Tinanoff N. Dental caries risk assessment and prevention. Dent Clin North Am 1995;39(4):709–19.
93. Fontana M, Zero DT. Assessing patients' caries risk. JADA 2006;137(9):1231–9.
94. Bader JD, Brown JP. Dilemmas in caries diagnosis. JADA 1993;124(6):48–50.
95. Dodds MW. Dilemmas in caries diagnosis: applications to current practice and need for research. J Dent Educ 1993;57(6):433–8.
96. van Dorp CS, Exterkate RA, ten Cate JM. The effect of dental probing on subsequent enamel demineralization. ASDC J Dent Child 1998;55(5):343–7.
97. American Dental Association. U.S. Food and Drug Administration. The selection of patients for dental radiographic examinations. Revised 2004. Available at: www.ada.org/prof/resources/topics/radiography.asp. Accessed January 12, 2008
98. Zandoná AF, Zero DT. Diagnostic tools for early caries detection. JADA 2006; 137(12):1675–84.
99. Bader JD, Shugars DA. A systematic review of the performance of a laser fluorescence device for detecting caries. JADA 2004;135(10):1413–26.

Evidence-Based Caries, Risk Assessment, and Treatment

Margherita Fontana, DDS, PhD[a],*, Douglas A. Young, DDS, MS, MBA[b],
Mark S. Wolff, DDS, PhD[c]

KEYWORDS

• Evidence base • Dental caries • Risk assessment
• Treatment • Management

Dental caries is a dietary and host-modified biofilm disease process, transmissible early in life that, if left untreated, will cause destruction of dental hard tissues. If allowed to progress, the disease will result in the development of caries lesions on tooth surfaces, which initially are noncavitated (eg, white spots), and eventually can progress to cavitation. The "medical model," where the etiologic disease-driving agents are balanced against protective factors, in combination with risk assessment, offers the possibility of patient-centered disease prevention and management before there is irreversible damage done to the teeth. This article discusses how to use evidence supporting risk assessment and management strategies for the caries process.

WHAT IS EVIDENCE-BASED DENTISTRY?

Evidence-based dentistry (EBD) is defined by American Dental Association (ADA) as an approach to oral health care that requires clinical decision-making based on the judicious integration of systematic assessments of clinically relevant scientific evidence relating to the patient's oral and medical condition and history; the dentist's clinical expertise; and the patient's treatment needs and preferences.[1] Of the three determinants listed above, the use of current science by the clinician in the decision-making process is critical. Patients expect health professionals to keep current in their field and they rely on these professionals to think critically through available diagnostic and treatment options, to help patient's make informed decisions about

[a] Department of Preventive and Community Dentistry, Indiana University School of Dentistry, 1121 W. Michigan Street, Room DS-406, Indianapolis, IN 46202, USA
[b] Department of Dental Practice, University of the Pacific, San Francisco, 2155 Webster Street, Room. 400, San Francisco, CA 94115, USA
[c] Department of Cariology and Comprehensive Care, New York University College of Dentistry, 345 East 24th Street (MC9480), New York, NY 10010, USA
* Corresponding author.
E-mail address: mfontan@iupui.edu (M. Fontana).

Dent Clin N Am 53 (2009) 149–161
doi:10.1016/j.cden.2008.10.003
0011-8532/08/$ – see front matter © 2009 Elsevier Inc. All rights reserved.

their health. On the other hand, dental treatments offered by a clinician do rely heavily on the dentist's "clinical expertise." However, if this is done without consideration of current available science and evidence, clinical treatment choices may be limited only to what "works well in my hands," or on information that has been passed from one practitioner to another. The public has the reasonable expectation that a health professional has a significantly high level of current scientific knowledge in his or her field. Even with this public expectation, the movement toward evidence-based medicine is only a decade and a half old,[2] and the movement toward evidence-based dentistry is even newer.

As logical as EBD sounds when it comes to the "medical" management of the disease of dental caries, its translation into practice has not been universally or enthusiastically embraced by all dental practitioners. There are many plausible explanations for this, but an important one to consider is that the findings of available scientific evidence may challenge and question current clinical practice. Some practitioners may sometimes struggle with the adoption of new concepts that challenge practice as they know it, even when they have strong clinical research evidence. An example of this is the fact that practitioners have been slow to adopt sealant therapy to protect susceptible pits and fissures of posterior teeth and arrest the progression of early caries lesions, despite the fact that there is very strong evidence to support their use.[3,4]

That being said, we need to acknowledge that maintaining an evidence-based knowledge on every aspect of dental practice can be an overwhelming and daunting task for any dental professional. The volume of information is substantial, frequently difficult to locate, and even more difficult to separate appropriate science from unreliable information. It is frequent that the information found is contradictory and the clinician is left to decide which evidence is more credible. In addition, a large portion of the dental workforce worldwide was not trained to critically search or evaluate research findings. Thus, clinicians are uncertain how to incorporate evidence-based practice into their everyday practice model. Baelum[5] suggested that dental schools, continuing professional education, and organized dentistry have very important roles in helping clinicians make sense of available evidence, either through educating practitioners in the techniques of EBD or in providing repositories of best practices based on sound evidence.

LEVELS OF SCIENTIFIC EVIDENCE: HOW MUCH IS ENOUGH?

Searching the existing literature to locate the best evidence and determining the quality of the evidence available is not as difficult as translating this evidence into changes in clinical guidelines. Shekelle and colleagues[6] developed a process for the development of guidelines that have been used within Europe and North America. This process starts with classifying evidence. Their suggested levels of evidence classification scheme, and strength of the evidence for a clinical recommendation, was based on the likelihood that evidence is susceptible to bias (eg, nature of the evidence), and thus, based on the effectiveness of studies by study design. In their scheme, the highest level of evidence is given to evidence derived from meta-analysis and systematic reviews of randomized, controlled trials (which implies that more than one trial is available on the topic), followed in a downward direction by: "evidence from at least one randomized controlled trial; evidence from at least one controlled study without randomization; evidence from at least one other type of quasi-experimental study; evidence from non-experimental descriptive studies, such as comparative studies, correlation studies, and case-control studies," and finally to "evidence from expert committee reports or opinions or clinical experience of respected authorities, or both."

The ultimate goal of this process is the translation of research findings into evidence-based clinical recommendations or interventions. To accomplish this, it is very important not only to look at the strength of the evidence, as described above, but also at how applicable the research finding is to the populations of interest (eg, in other words, is the evidence generalizable or applicable?). In addition, it is also necessary to determine the cost of the intervention, and the feasibility of the intervention in the context of the existing health care system. The intervention must finally be evaluated as to how it interferes or interfaces with the current beliefs and values of those who will use it (eg, how acceptable will it be to the practitioner?).[6]

In dentistry generally, and caries management particularly, it is surprising how few studies, representing a high strength of evidence (ie, meta-analyses or systematic reviews of randomized, controlled clinical trials), exist for many of our daily intervention choices. However, limited or few apex-level evidence studies for many of the interventions that are currently available to manage dental caries does not mean that dentistry should not develop practice guidelines based on the best current evidence available for their use. If dentistry does not develop appropriate evidence-based guidelines, these interventions may be incorporated in practice in a random, disorganized and possibly incorrect manner. Recent examples of such evidence-based practice guidelines are those developed by the ADA for in-office professionally applied topical fluorides[1] and for use of dental sealants.[3] These guidelines are based on significant volumes of high-level research.

One of the most complete evidence-based reviews of many aspects of caries risk assessment and management was done in 2001 for the Consensus Conference on Caries Management, sponsored in the National Institutes of Health. Multiple systematic reviews were performed on caries detection and diagnosis, risk assessment, and a variety of management strategies both for adult and pediatric populations. The reviews and presentations were compiled and published in 2001 in the *Journal of Dental Education*, together with a summary consensus statement,[7] and still are an excellent source for evidence-based caries management information.

TRADITIONAL CARIES MANAGEMENT: THE CASE OF MINIMAL EVIDENCE FOR CARIES THERAPY

Between the years 1869 and 1915, Greene V. Black published a series of papers and texts on dental materials and preparation or restoration techniques that changed dentistry. Though many current investigators have credited or criticized these tenants for overly aggressive preparations and restorations in modern dentistry,[8,9] G.V. Black was the first dentist to propose treating dental caries using minimal intervention, based on the knowledge and materials available at that time. Therefore, Black was indeed using, for his time, an evidence-based approach to dealing with the nineteenth century understanding of dental caries. During that time, the exact cause of dental caries was an unknown, cavity preparations were designed at the will of the operating dentist with no science, and dental amalgam alloy was frequently formulated by the dentist and had little standardization. These inconsistencies resulted in materials and restorations demonstrating poor performance. G.V. Black, a dentist of considerable experience and observational skills, noted the frequent failure of dental amalgam restorations with recurrent caries at the corroded margins of the restorations. Patients were observed to develop caries on virgin approximal surfaces because of the stagnation of food in these uncleansable areas. Patients were also observed to develop caries around occlusal restorations that failed to include susceptible pits and fissures.

Black[10,11] wrote a series of papers that addressed the problems of caries at the margins of restorations and tooth restorations.[12] These papers represented the earliest workbooks on quality operative dentistry of that era, and these papers were based on the best knowledge available. Though not a single controlled, clinical research project was published to develop these criteria, they represented the personal observations and opinions of an expert, the lowest level of research credibility.

Black described the placement of the outer enamel margins in "self cleansable areas" so that they terminated in regions less susceptible to recurrent caries. Black wrote, "Certainly that portion near the proximate contact... is most liable to be attacked; and the liability diminishes as we recede from that point... it is to cut the enamel margins from lines that are not self cleansing to lines that are self-cleansing," and "When a cavity has occurred in the occluding surface of a molar, the dentist prepares for filling with the idea that the fissures in this part of the enamel have favored the occurrence of the cavity. For this reason the fissures and grooves adjoining the cavity, even though not decayed, are cut away to such a point as seems to give opportunity for a smooth, even finish of the margins of the filling. This is done as a prevention of future recurrence of decay...." This led to the now infamous term "extension for prevention," which could be summed up as "...the removal of the enamel margin by cutting from a point of greater liability to a point of lesser liability to recurrence of caries...." Furthermore, he developed an amalgam alloy less likely to corrode and suffer marginal breakdown, whose formula remained essentially unchanged until the 1970s, when high copper-silver amalgams were introduced.[13] In addition, he developed standard and meticulous placement techniques for dental amalgam that used proper isolation. "...Restorations of cohesive gold and amalgam... require the application of the rubber dam... The student or dentist who earnestly desires to give the best service will, when in doubt, apply the rubber dam."

This remained the state of dental education and clinical practice until the 1950s, 60s, and 70s. During this period of time, several events occurred that allowed the improvement of dental amalgams and the introduction of bonded restorations. Amalgams were improved by the development of a process whereby the amalgam alloy was triturated with the ideal quantity of mercury, known as the Eames Technique.[14] Clinical research was performed to determine the effect that higher copper-content alloys, having less creep and marginal breakdown, had on improving the alloy longevity,[15–17] but not to determine if these improvements reduced the rates of new or recurrent caries development. Clinical research demonstrated that smaller preparations displayed less material break down, but not that they were less likely to develop recurrent caries.[18] These breakthroughs each led to changes in preparation design and restorations that were smaller and more effective, but not less likely to experience recurrent or new caries. In fact, the above studies report recurrent caries as a rationale for failure of the restoration!

The scientific advances in bonding resulted in the greatest change in operative dentistry since the publications of Black. In 1955, Buonocore[19] described a technique for etching the enamel surface to improve retention of restorative materials and, shortly thereafter, Bowen submitted a patent entitled a "Dental filling material comprising vinyl silane treated fused silica and a binder consisting of BIS phenol and glycidyl acrylic" that enabled the restoration of a tooth with a tooth colored plastic, better known today as Bis-GMA. These two developments have resulted in the possibility of better tooth conservation or minimally invasive surgical dentistry. For example, the historic rationale for removal of an intact groove was prevention of future caries. The concern of future caries in the groove is easily dealt with by placement of a sealant, a technique well documented to prevent and arrest caries.[3,4] In a sense, this is a similar concept to Black's extension for prevention but uses the advantages of the relatively new restorative materials without the need for surgical excision and extension.

The traditional surgical method for treatment of dental caries will not eliminate the disease.[20] In reality, the fact that the existence of recent restorations is the greatest indicator of risk for the development of new lesions[7,21] only proves that the act of surgically treating the caries lesion does little to reduce the risk of developing the next lesion. Interestingly, a recent systematic review found no difference in pulpal vitality, symptoms, and longevity of restorations, irrespective of whether removal of infected tissue in a deep cavity had been minimal or complete.[22] Therefore, evidence is challenging our current views of restorative dentistry.

CARIES MANAGEMENT BY RISK ASSESSMENT: HOW MUCH EVIDENCE IS NEEDED?

In contrast to the traditional management of dental caries based on surgical restoration of tooth damage alone, current management strategies explore treating dental caries based on an individual risk assessment of the patient (because each patient presents with their own unique set of pathologic and protective factors).[23–31] Caries management by risk assessment (CAMBRA) was developed to promote the clinical management philosophy in which the caries disease process is managed following the medical model. This involves an evaluation of the etiologic and protective factors and establishment of the risk for future disease (risk assessment), followed by development of a patient-centered evidence-based caries management plan.[32] The infectious-caries disease paradigm is based on the fact that dental caries is caused by identifiable bacterial pathogens that are part of a complex biofilm, of which mutans streptococci[33] and lactobacilli have been extensively studied. These cariogenic bacteria thrive in acidic environments, while producing acids themselves, altering the environment to favor their own viability.[34] These are extensively modulated by environmental changes, with a sucrose-rich diet being an important risk factor. These pathogens can colonize emerging tooth surfaces in children, transmitted for example from mother to child,[35–42] as well as from tooth to tooth by improper use of the dental explorer,[43] although the clinical implications of this latter process are less well understood.

In this disease model, carious lesions can be thought of as visible "signs" on the teeth of a chronic, potentially progressive disease process resulting from the interaction between the bacterial biofilm ecology and the conditions in the oral environment. When the active disease is diagnosed early, these bacteria can be chemotherapeutically targeted, as would any active bacterial infection in the body. The difficulty is that the pathogenic cariogenic biofilm is composed by bacteria that are part of our normal oral biofilm in an altered distribution, and not external pathogens. Thus, controlling and managing this biofilm becomes a complicated medical challenge for which more effective and less compliance-dependent treatments are still necessary for at-risk groups. If the infectious disease is allowed to progress and demineralization is not countered with remineralization, cavitations will result.[29] Once cavitation through enamel allows bacterial to invade the dentin, minimally invasive restoration may be appropriate and necessary.[44] The ultimate goal is to prevent and manage the disease process before tooth cavitation is allowed to occur, whereas traditional restorative methods intervene only after advanced disease destruction (cavitation) has taken place.

Appropriate CAMBRA management depends on the stage of the disease process and subsequent severity of damage to the dentition.[45,46] It includes the consideration of strategies that delay and reduce the early transmission of cariogenic microflora, control the infection, prevent or remineralize the early manifestations of the disease on the teeth, and appropriately manage the more advanced stages of tooth demineralization and cavitation. CAMBRA supports the use of chemical remineralization of early pre-cavitated lesions and sealing of occlusal noncavitated lesions,[3,4,47] along with tooth-preserving and minimally invasive restorative techniques (minimal surgical intervention) when deemed necessary in treating cavitated lesions.

The caries risk marker with the strongest evidence of correlation to future disease from the literature is still, unfortunately, past caries experience.[7,21] This can be measured clinically in many ways (eg, the presence and number of noncavitated "white-spot" lesions, presence and number of recent restorations, radiographic enamel or dentin lesions, and cavitations). Many other risk factors and risk indicators have been studied in a variety of population groups, but results have been varied. However, an assessment of the caries etiologic factors (eg, plaque, diet) and protective factors (eg, exposure to fluoride, adequate salivary flow) can help inform the individualized causes for dental caries disease in a patient and help drive the development of a patient-centered, evidence-based management plan (**Fig. 1**).

When searching the literature for evidence-based clinical recommendations in managing and preventing dental caries, the highest level of evidence and strongest recommendations based on systematic reviews of randomized, controlled clinical trials can be found for fluorides[1,48–53] and sealants.[3,54,55] The results of these research reviews worldwide have been unambiguous and consistent in their support of the

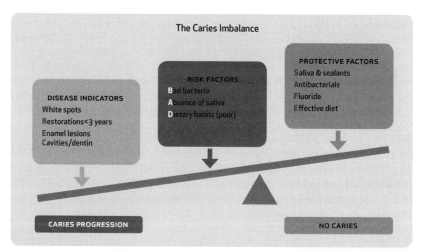

Fig. 1. The caries "imbalance." The balance amongst disease indicators, risk factors, and protective factors determines whether dental caries progresses, halts, or reverses. "Cavities/dentin" refers to frank cavities or lesions to the dentin by radiograph. "Restorations <3 years" means restorations placed in the previous 3 years. This figure has been updated from previous versions of the "caries balance," with the very important addition of the disease indicators. If these indicators are present, they weigh heavily on the side of predicting caries progression unless therapeutic intervention is performed. The leading letters that help to remember the imbalance (WREC, BAD, SAFE) have been added, as well as "sealants" as a protective factor. "Dietary habits (poor)" indicates frequent ingestion of fermentable carbohydrates (greater than three times daily between meals). (*From* Featherstone JDB, Domejean-Orliaguet S, Jenson L, et al. Caries risk assessment in practice for age 6 through adult. J Calif Dent Assoc 2007;35:705. Reprinted from the California Dental Association; with permission.)

efficacy of fluoride as a caries-preventive measure. Therefore, it is critical that caries treatment guidelines and individualized caries management strategies include these effective strategies. However, even in practices using risk-based prevention of caries, fluoride is often not used in an optimal manner. For example, Bader and colleagues[56] reported that in a group of 15 volunteer private practices using risk-based prevention of dental caries, fluoride-intervention modalities were only used in 63% of identified high caries-risk patients and 32% of identified moderate caries-risk patients. This is in contrast to ADA recommendations published in 2006 for in-office topical fluoride applications.[1] Bader and colleagues[56] found practices very willing to perform caries risk assessment and caries risk-based prevention, and concluded this was indeed a feasible approach in practice today. However, they called for "more intensive exposure to fluorides in preventive treatment for patients at elevated risk of developing caries."

Other than fluoride and sealants, a wide variety of strategies have been used and proposed in the literature, either for the individual or population-based management of dental caries. These include, among others: use of antimicrobials (eg, chlorhexidine, xylitol, ozone, and others), dietary counseling or modification, oral hygiene, calcium-based strategies, and so forth. In general, the evidence supporting these additional strategies is much more varied and in some cases conflicting or derived from lower strength of evidence. In other words, there are many studies relating to individual products used in the treatment of dental caries but very few randomized, controlled clinical trials using a risk-based approach or comparing multiple products and strategies in varied populations. Regardless, in some cases these additional strategies or products may remain clinically relevant and useful in selected patient populations, based on best evidence currently available.

The objective of this article is not to review the literature on every aspect of dental caries risk assessment and management. This has been done by others.[7,57] The irrefutable effectiveness of many of these known caries management strategies (eg, calcium-based strategies, chlorhexidine, and others) still is discouraging, and in many cases the evidence is insufficient to permit the formulation of evidence-based guidelines. Yet the concept of providing interventions based on the caries risk of a patient has increasing support in dentistry worldwide.[58–60] As stated by Bader and colleagues[57] "typically, the discussion is focused on classifying individuals' risk, with the assumption being made that once the classification is made, appropriate preventive therapy will follow, which presumably will prove to be efficacious... It is likely that the infrequent appearance of specific treatment recommendations and efficacy estimates for children and adults by risk category in the recent literature is due at least in part to a lack of knowledge of the efficacy of preventive interventions among individuals with specific caries risk classifications."

An example of how evidence is sometimes difficult to digest by the clinician is the evidence available on two caries management strategies and products available in the United States market: xylitol and casein-based products. There have been many reviews written on the use of xylitol for caries prevention and management, and almost all of those reviews strongly favor the use of xylitol to reduce mutans streptococci bacterial counts[61,62] and acid production.[63,64] In a 2001 systematic review, Hayes[65] concluded that xylitol may significantly decrease the incidence of dental caries. However, a 2003 systematic review concluded that the evidence for the use of sorbitol or xylitol in chewing gum for caries prevention was inconclusive[66] How is the clinician to interpret these mixed data?

Another such example is the use of casein derivatives. Although a lot of work has been presented to suggest that casein derivatives are effective in caries prevention,[67–70] there have been publications that have found no effect[71,72] and a recent systematic review concluded that "the quantity and quality of clinical trial evidence are insufficient to make conclusions regarding the long-term effectiveness of casein derivatives, specifically CPP-ACP, in preventing caries in vivo and treating dentin hypersensitivity or dry mouth."[73]

Ultimately, the question that the clinician will ask is what can be safely incorporated into practice. Use of evidence-based recommendations by organized dentistry[1,3] are excellent sources of information and guidance. Systematic reviews are also a great source of information. Even if the review finds that there are few studies or they are conflicting, they can help the reader locate important references on the specific topic that may help inform the dentist's decision. It is, however, very important to stress that the absence of strong studies to support a particular intervention, or inconclusive results when reviewing it, does not necessarily mean that the intervention does not work. It means that dentists need to be aware of the current level of evidence supporting the intervention (ie, to determine how reliable are the results up to now), how the intervention may compare to or affect other available stronger evidence-based intervention choices (ie, so that interventions that are known to work well are not substitued for those we are less sure about), and that the guidelines on the intervention's use may change in the future pending the availability of stronger evidence. Most critically, understanding the strength (or weakness) of the evidence to support many treatment recommendations for dental caries urges us to consider therapeutic choices that are as noninvasive and destructive as possible, to avoid doing irreversible damage. It also urges us to consider, when considering the incorporation of newer strategies that seem promising but for which the level of evidence supporting them is lower, to use these newer strategies, if so desired, to supplement well-known interventions, rather than substituting them.

OBSTACLES FOR EVIDENCE: RANDOMIZED, CONTROLLED CARIES MANAGEMENT CLINICAL TRIALS

Why aren't there more randomized clinical trials on risk-based management of caries? The design and implementation of a clinical trial to detect clinically and statistically significant differences between multiple treatment interventions based on risk, is extremely expensive and time-consuming. Randomized clinical trials for dental caries on human subjects require many years for caries lesions to form and progress to cavitation, which is still the only acceptable outcome measurement. In addition to various logistical problems, there are obvious ethical issues with such a trial. Large sample sizes are required because of difficulties with research subject retention and long-term follow up, especially if differences between treatments under study may be subtle. The conclusions of these studies are normally difficult to generalize and are, therefore, only relevant to the population group that was studied. For example, if a study focused on children (this is commonly done because they are easy to follow while in school settings), the conclusions may not be easily generalized to other age groups. Thus, if therapeutic approaches tested in children are suggested to be of use in adults, it is with much less certainty and thus, evidence strength. Because of the problems inherent in such trials, there is, in general, "comparatively little information available describing the efficacy of caries management and prevention interventions among high risk individuals." Furthermore, information on the efficacy of these interventions on noncavitated lesions is inconsistent because, until recently, there have not been established criteria to assess these that would allow study comparisons.[57]

Unfortunately, a dearth of randomized clinical trials affects the conclusions of systematic reviews and meta-analyses on the subject of caries management and prevention. The systematic review and meta-analysis are based on the availability of randomized, controlled trials of similar design. When such studies are not available or are few, or study results are not always in agreement, results of the systematic reviews are many times inconclusive, meaning that a clear decision could not be reached. Furthermore, some products used to treat and prevent caries in the United States are not specifically Food and Drug Administration-approved to treat caries, yet the off label use of some of these products for dental caries has been demonstrated and, thus, they are routinely used by dentists. If patients are already using these products for caries management there is, obviously, less incentive for industry to spend large sums of money on clinical trials. In addition, there is a great demand for new treatment products to treat dental caries and many of these products are coming from new start-up companies with insufficient resources to fund robust, clinical trials.

SUMMARY

The methods used for treating dental caries in practice today remain largely focused on the use of surgical tooth restoration alone (ie, restorative treatment), without consistent and individualized consideration of the underlying disease process for each patient. But, there is no evidence that restorative care effectively prevents or manages the dental caries disease process. Clinical trials to provide clear evidence regarding the effectiveness of various risk-based caries interventions are insufficient to permit the formulation of definitive guidelines. Thus, the clinician is left with two choices: continue using the outdated traditional restorative-only approach based on irreversible procedures, or use nondestructive risk-based caries management strategies using best scientific evidence available. The latter choice is the one that the scientific community has been encouraging the profession to embrace. Except for fluorides and sealants, evidence for other caries management strategies is less strong and more controversial, so dentists are encouraged not to incorporate these strategies as a replacement of higher evidence strategies, but to supplement them, if so desired, with a clear understanding of the evidence indicating they may be effective. It is clear that the search for more effective and practical therapeutic approaches for the management of patients at risk for dental caries needs to continue, as does the search for stronger evidence for available treatment strategies and choices. In summary, the goal of ideal evidence-based patient care is to always select the therapeutic option that is supported by the highest level of evidence and that is applicable, feasible, and acceptable to the particular dentist-patient team.

REFERENCES

1. American Dental Association Council on Scientific Affairs. Professionally applied topical fluoride: evidence-based clinical recommendations. J Am Dent Assoc 2006;137(8):1151–9.
2. Evidence-Based Medicine Working Group. Evidence-based medicine. A new approach to teaching the practice of medicine. JAMA 1992;268(17):2420–5.
3. Beauchamp J, Caufield PW, Crall JJ, et al. Evidence-based clinical recommendations for the use of pit-and-fissure sealants. A report of the American Dental Association Council on Scientific Affairs. J Am Dent Assoc 2008;139:257–68.
4. Griffin SO, Oong E, Kohn W, et al. The effectiveness of sealants in managing caries lesions. J Dent Res 2008;87(2):169–74.

5. Baelum V, Kidd OFE. Clinical decision making: technical solutions to biological problems or evidence-based caries management? In: Dental caries. The disease and its clinical management. Blackwell Munksgaard Ltd; 2008. p. 459–71.

6. Shekelle PG, Steven HW, Martin E, et al. Clinical guidelines: developing guidelines. BMJ 1999;318(7183):593–6.

7. National Institutes of Health Consensus Development Conference Statement. NIH consensus development conference on diagnosis and management of dental caries throughout life. Bethesda, MD, March 26–28, 2001. Conference papers. J Dent Educ 2001;65(10):1162–8.

8. Chalmers JM. Minimal intervention dentistry: part 1. Strategies for addressing the new caries challenge in older patients. J Can Dent Assoc 2006;72(5):427–33.

9. Mount GJ. Minimal intervention dentistry: rationale of cavity design. Oper Dent 2003;28(1):92–9.

10. Black GV. Management of enamel margins. Dent Cosmos 1891;33:1–14 [85–100, 440–7].

11. Black GV. The effect of oxidation on cut alloys for dental amalgams. Dent Cosmos 1896;38:43–8.

12. Black GV. A work on operative dentistry volume two, technical procedures in filling teeth. Chicago: Medico-Dental Publishing Co; 1908.

13. Anusavice KJ. Phillips' science of dental materials. 11th edition. St. Louis (MO): Saunders; 2003.

14. Eames WB. Preparation and condensation of amalgam with a low mercuryalloy ratio. J Am Dent Assoc 1959;58(4):78–83.

15. Osborne JW, Norman RD. 13-year clinical assessment of 10 amalgam alloys. Dent Mater 1990;6(3):189–94.

16. Letzel H, van 't Hof MA, Marshall GW, et al. The influence of the amalgam alloy on the survival of amalgam restorations: a secondary analysis of multiple controlled clinical trials. J Dent Res 1997;76(11):1787–98.

17. Mahler DB. The high-copper dental amalgam alloys. J Dent Res 1997;76(1):537–41.

18. Osborne JW, Gale EN. Relationship of restoration width, tooth position, and alloy to fracture at the margins of 13- to 14-year-old amalgams. J Dent Res 1990;69(9):1599–601.

19. Buonocore MG. A simple method of increasing the adhesion of acrylic filling materials to enamel surfaces. J Dent Res 1955;34(6):849–53.

20. Featherstone JDB, Gansky SA, Hoover CI, et al. A randomized clinical trial of caries management by risk assessment. Caries Res 2005;39:295 [abstract 25].

21. Zero D, Fontana M, Lennon AM. Clinical applications and outcomes of using indicators of risk in caries management. J Dent Educ 2001;65(10):1126–32.

22. Ricketts DNJ, Kidd EAM, Innes N, et al. Complete or ultraconservative removal of decayed tissue in unfilled teeth. Cochrane Database Syst Rev 2006.

23. Anderson MH, Molvar MP, Powell LV. Treating dental caries as an infectious disease. Oper Dent 1991;16(1):21–8.

24. Anderson MH, Bales DJ, Omnell K-A. Modern management of dental caries: the cutting edge is not the dental bur. J Am Dent Assoc 1993;124:37–44.

25. Anderson MH. Changing paradigms in caries management. Curr Opin Dent 1992;2:157–62.

26. Anusavice KJ. Treatment regimens in preventive and restorative dentistry. J Am Dent Assoc 1995;126(6):727–43.

27. Pitts NB. Patient caries status in the context of practical, evidence-based management of the initial caries lesion. J Dent Educ 1997;61:895–905.

28. Suddick RP, Dodds MWJ. Caries activity estimates and implications: insights into risk versus activity. J Dent Educ 1997;61:876–84.
29. Featherstone JD. The science and practice of caries prevention. J Am Dent Assoc 2000;131(7):887–99.
30. Young DA. New caries detection technologies and modern caries management: Merging the strategies. Gen Dent 2002;50(4):320–31.
31. Fontana M, Zero DT. Assessing patients' caries risk. J Am Dent Assoc 2006; 137(9):1231–9.
32. Young DA, Featherstone JD, Roth JR. Curing the silent epidemic: caries management in the 21st century and beyond. J Calif Dent Assoc 2007;35(10):681–5.
33. Loesche WJ. Role of Streptococcus mutans in human dental decay. FEMS Microbiol Rev 1986;50:353–80.
34. Marsh P. Dental diseases—are these examples of ecological catastrophes? Int J Dent Hyg 2006;4(Suppl 1):3–10.
35. Caufield PW, Cutter GR, Dasanayake AP. Initial acquisition of mutans streptococci by infants: evidence for a discrete window of infectivity. J Dent Res 1993; 72(1):37–45.
36. Wan AK, Seo WK, Purdie DM, et al. Oral colonization of Streptococcus mutans in six-month-old predentate infants. J Dent Res 2001;80(12):2060–5.
37. Wan AK, Seow WK, Walsh LJ, et al. Association of Streptococcus mutans infection and oral developmental nodules in pre-dentate infants. J Dent Res 2001; 80(10):1945–8.
38. Mattos-Graner RO, Li Y, Caufield PW, et al. Genotypic diversity of mutans streptococci in Brazilian nursery children suggests horizontal transmission. J Clin Microbiol 2001; 39(6):2313–6.
39. Mattos-Graner RO, Corrêa MS, Latorre MR, et al. Mutans streptococci oral colonization in 12–30-month-old Brazilian children over a one-year follow-up period. J Public Health Dent 2001;61(3):161–7.
40. Kohler B, Andreen I, Jonsson B. The earlier the colonization by mutans streptococci, the higher the caries prevalence at 4 years of age. Oral Microbiol Immunol 1988;3(1):14–7.
41. Davey AL, Rogers AH. Multiple types of the bacterium Streptococcus mutans in the human mouth and their intra-family transmission. Arch Oral Biol 1984;29(6):453–60.
42. van Loveren C, Buijs JF, ten Cate JM. Similarity of bacteriocin activity profiles of mutans streptococci within the family when the children acquire the strains after the age of 5. Caries Res 2000;34(6):481–5.
43. Loesche WJ, Svanberg ML, Pape HR. Intraoral transmission of Streptococcus mutans by a dental explorer. J Dent Res 1979;58(8):1765–70.
44. Featherstone JD, Cutress TW, Rodgers BE, et al. Remineralization of artificial caries-like lesions in vivo by a self-administered mouthrinse or paste. Caries Res 1982;16(3):235–42.
45. Ramos-Gomez FJ, Crall J, Gansky ST, et al. Caries risk assessment appropriate for the age 1 visit (infants and toddlers). J Calif Dent Assoc 2007;35(10):687–702.
46. Jenson L, Budenz AW, Featherstone JDB, et al. Clinical protocols for caries management by risk assessment. J Calif Dent Assoc 2007;35(10):714–23.
47. Oong EM, et al. The effect of dental sealants on bacteria levels in caries lesions: a review of the evidence. J Am Dent Assoc 2008;139(3):271–8 [quiz: 357–8].
48. Marinho V, Higgins J, Logan S, et al. Fluoride gels for preventing dental caries in children and adolescents. Cochrane Database Syst Rev 2002.
49. Marinho V, Higgins J, Logan S, et al. Fluoride mouthrinses for preventing dental caries in children and adolescents. Cochrane Database Syst Rev 2003.

50. Marinho V, Higgins J, Logan S, et al. Fluoride toothpastes for preventing dental caries in children and adolescents. Cochrane Database Syst Rev 2003.
51. Marinho V, Higgins J, Logan S, et al. Fluoride varnishes for preventing dental caries in children and adolescents. Cochrane Database Syst Rev 2002.
52. Marinho V, Higgins J, Sheiham A, et al. One topical fluoride (toothpastes, or mouthrinses, or gels, or varnishes) versus another for preventing dental caries in children and adolescents. Cochrane Database Syst Rev 2004.
53. Benson P, Parkin N, Millett D, et al. Fluorides for the prevention of white spots on teeth during fixed brace treatment. Cochrane Database Syst Rev 2004.
54. Ahovuo-Saloranta A, Hiiri A, Nordblad A, et al. Pit and fissure sealants for preventing dental decay in the permanent teeth of children and adolescents. Cochrane Database Syst Rev 2004.
55. Hiiri A, Ahovuo-Saloranta A, Nordblad A, et al. Pit and fissure sealants versus fluoride varnishes for preventing dental decay in children and adolescents. Cochrane Database Syst Rev 2006.
56. Bader J, DA S, Kennedy J, et al. A pilot study of risk-based prevention in provate practice. J Am Dent Assoc 2003;134:1195–202.
57. Bader J, Shugars D, Bonito A. A systematic review of selected caries prevention and management methods. Community Dent Oral Epidemiol 2001;29:399–411.
58. American Dental Association, C.o.A., Prevention, and Interprofessional Relations. Caries diagnosis and risk assessment: a review of preventive strategies and management. J Am Dent Assoc 1995;126(Suppl):1s–24s.
59. Pitts N. Risk assessment and caries prediction. J Dent Educ 1998;62:762–70.
60. Featherstone JD. The caries balance: the basis for caries management by risk assessment. Oral Health Prev Dent 2004;(2 Suppl 1):259–64.
61. Soderling E, Isokangas P, Pienihakkinen K, et al. Influence of maternal xylitol consumption on mother-child transmission of mutans streptococci: 6-year follow-up. Caries Res 2001;35:173–7.
62. Haresaku S, Hanioka T, Tsutsui A, et al. Long-term effect of xylitol gum use on mutans streptococci in adults. Caries Res 2007;41:198–203.
63. Twetman S, Stecksen-Blicks C. Effect of xylitol-containing chewing gums on lactic acid production in dental plaque from caries active pre-school children. Oral Health Prev Dent 2003;1:195–9.
64. Holgerson P, Sjostrom I, Stecksen-Blicks C, et al. Dental plaque formation and salivary mutans streptococci in schoolchildren after use of xylitol-containing chewing gum. Int J Paediatr Dent 2007;17:79–85.
65. Hayes C. The effect of non-cariogenic sweeteners on the prevention of dental caries: a review of the evidence. J Dent Educ 2001;65(10):1106–9.
66. Lingström P, Holm A-K, Mejàre I, et al. Dietary factors in the prevention of dental caries: a systematic review. Acta Odontol Scand 2003;61(6):331–40.
67. Reynolds EC, Cain CJ, Webber FL, et al. Anticariogenicity of calcium phosphate complexes of tryptic casein phosphopeptides in the rat. J Dent Res 1995;74(6):1272–9.
68. Reynolds EC. Remineralization of enamel subsurface lesions by casein phosphopeptide-stabilized calcium phosphate solutions. J Dent Res 1997;76(9):1587–95.
69. Rose R. Binding characteristics of Streptococcus mutans for calcium and casein phosphopeptide. Caries Res 2000;34(5):427–31.
70. Rose R. Effects of an anticariogenic casein phosphopeptide on calcium diffusion in streptococcal model dental plaques. Arch Oral Biol 2000;45(7):569–75.

71. Itthagarun A, King N, Yiu C, et al. The effect of chewing gums containing calcium phosphates on the remineralization of artificial caries-like lesions in situ. Caries Res 2005;39(3):251–4.
72. Hay K, Thomson W. A clinical trial of the anticaries efficacy of casein derivatives complexed with calcium phosphate in patients with salivary gland dysfunction. Oral Surg Oral Med Oral Pathol Oral Radiol Endod 2002;93(3):271–5.
73. Azarpazhooh A, Limeback H. Clinical efficacy of casein derivatives. A systematic review of the literature. J Am Dent Assoc 2008;139(7):915–24.

Index

Note: Page numbers of article titles are in **boldface** type.

A

Abutment tooth, for single tooth replacement, attached keratinized tissue and, 102
    clinical crown for, 102
    considerations for, 99–102
    endodontic therapy and, 102
    periodontal attachment loss and, 101
    periodontal stability of, 100–101
    restorative margin position/gengival margin, 101–102
Adhesives, and resins, in dentinal hypersensitivity, 54–55
Alendronate, 23, 24
Amalgam, versus composite, in restoration of posterior teeth, in clinical practice, **71–76**
American Association of Oral and Maxillofacial Surgeons, age-related third-molar study,
    78–81
    parameters of care, 77–78
    third-molar clinical trial of, 81–91
    "White Paper on third molar data," 91–93
American Dental Association, Center for Evidence-based Dentistry, 135
    Council on Scientific Affairs, 131, 135

B

Bisphosphonate-related osteonecrosis of jaws, 23–30

C

Calcium compounds, in dentinal hypersensitivity, 51
Caries, definition of, 132–133
    epidemiology of, 133
    evidence-based, risk assessment, and treatment, **149–161**
    management of, by risk assessment, 153–156
        randomized controlled clinical trials of, 156–157
    occlusal, retention of third molars and, 90–91
    pit-and-fissure sealants in prevention of, 133, 137–141
    risk of, assessment of, 141
    therapy of, minimal evidence for, 151–153
    traditional management of, 151–153
Cavity lining, and varnishes, under restorations, 50–51
Cavity preparations, corticosteroids and, 51
Cements, glass ionomer versus resin-based, conditions for placement of, 141

Dent Clin N Am 53 (2009) 163–168
doi:10.1016/S0011-8532(08)00116-X
0011-8532/08/$ – see front matter © 2009 Elsevier Inc. All rights reserved.

dental.theclinics.com